PRAISE FOR
FOUNTAIN OF YOUTH

"THE STRAIGHT SKINNY! Lose weight and get younger—what a bargain! The plan is healthy and easy to follow, and the book is packed with great information about health, vitamins, and longevity. Comic relief comes from Edita's frank and funny telling of her own diet travails and triumphs."
—*Woman's Day*

"I loved FOUNTAIN OF YOUTH. . . . [It was] very informative (the extensive research was obvious) and fun to read as well. Edita's style is entertaining and her expertise is quite impressive . . . an inspiration to baby boomers who thought they'd seen better days. . . . She makes healthy living fun, easy, and effective."
—**Pam Mycoskie, author of *Butter Busters*®**

"Nutrition and meal plans are two surefire roads to losing weight and achieving longevity. Edita Kaye has laid out a wonderful road map."
—**Dharma Singh Khalsa, M.D., coauthor of *Brain Longevity***

"FOUNTAIN OF YOUTH is the right book at the right time. We baby boomers have needed a book like this—and rarely do you find one that is practical, helpful, and inspirational all at the same time."
—**Gregory J.P. Godek, author of the bestsellers**
1001 Ways to Be Romantic **and** *Love—The Course They
Forgot to Teach You in School*

"Overflows with information and inspiration for anyone who wants to get more out of mid-life."
—**Greg Dougherty, editor in chief, *New Choices* magazine**

"Stop wishing for lost youth already—Edita Kaye's FOUNTAIN OF YOUTH makes it a reality! The author is living proof—she's been there, done it. Her sensible plan of action . . . makes it easier than you think to return to happier, healthier days."
—**Beverly Berwald, editor, *Longevity Journal***

"Edita Kaye offers the most delightful, practical, and completely usable tools to achieve your own FOUNTAIN OF YOUTH—greater health, beauty, and confidence in yourself!"
—**Leigh Taylor, actor**

"Wonderfully entertaining guide to staying and looking young. It's a perfect complement for anyone seeking rejuvenation."
—**Steven Pearlman, M.D.**

ALSO BY EDITA KAYE

Bone Builders™: The Complete Lowfat Cookbook Plus Calcium Health Guide

FOUNTAIN OF YOUTH

The Anti-Aging Weight-Loss Program

Edita Kaye

WARNER BOOKS

A Time Warner Company

Important: Please Read Carefully
The information, ideas, suggestions, and answers to questions in this book are not intended to substitute for the services of a physician. You should only undertake a health and wellness modification program in conjunction with the services of a qualified health professional. This book is intended as a reference guide only, not as a manual for self-treatment. If you suspect you have a medical problem or have questions, please talk to your health care professional. All the information here is based on research available at the time of this printing.

Copyright © 1998 by Fountain of Youth Group, Inc.
All rights reserved.
Warner Books, Inc., 1271 Avenue of the Americas, New York, NY 10020
Visit our Web site at
http://warnerbooks.com

 A Time Warner Company

Printed in the United States of America
First Trade Printing: March 1999
10 9 8 7 6 5 4 3 2 1

The Library of Congress has cataloged the hardcover edition as follows:
Library of Congress Cataloging-in-Publication Data
Kaye, Edita
    Fountain of youth : the anti-aging weight-loss program / Edita Kaye.
        p. cm.
    ISBN 0-446-52161-2
    1. Longevity. 2. Nutrition. 3. Weight loss. I. Title.
RA776.75.K38   1998
613'.0434—dc21   97-9598
                                                              CIP

ISBN 0-446-67470-2 (pbk.)

Book design and composition by L&G McRee
Cover design by Wendy Bass
Cover photo by Joanne Savio

Fountain of Youth
is dedicated to my four fantastic sisters
Marg, Wanda, Eva, and Ania

ACKNOWLEDGMENTS

Lots of people touched my life and my work. I would like to say a special
thanks to them.

Thank you to . . .

Mark for listening, encouraging, suggesting. A special man. A special
friend. A very special son.

Tamara for becoming my daughter for the second time.

Larry Kirshbaum for believing in me.

Susan Suffes, who started as my editor and became my friend.

Jessica Papin, my new editor, who sent me a note to nourish my spirit
when I most needed it.

Flamur Tonuzi, who made me a cover girl. Way to go!

Bonnie, my favorite blond and soulmate for giving me the gift of the
spirit that has made everything that follows possible.

Claudia, my newest friend, for walking ten thousand miles with me
and making the journey memorable.

Carol for the pleasant evenings and the cultural adventures.

Cory Dalton & David Galluzzo for keeping me beautiful.

Lillian Brady, who helped me paddle through the rough seas.

John Dologhan for his words. I was listening and I heard.

Kristin Frias for her warmth and for letting me visit with Alexander.

Martha Coulter for finding me a beautiful and serene home.

Mark Lawless for reading the fine print.

Joanne Savio for the best picture I ever had of myself.

Patrick Devlin for giving me an option I hadn't considered.

Jan Bialka & Cathy Planner for being such dedicated booksellers.

All the special folks at the St. John's County Public Library System for helping with research.

CONTENTS

My Personal Story

If there is anything natural and inevitable about the aging process, it cannot be known until the chains of our old beliefs are broken.

—DEEPAK CHOPRA

This book is my own personal story. I write these words twelve years younger and twenty pounds thinner than I was ninety days ago. I turned back the clock. I lightened the scale. I believe I have found the fountain of youth. And when you read my story, I know you will believe it too.

A few short months ago, like so many of my friends, facing the big forty or fifty, I was frightened of getting older. I spent hours examining the first bulge of jowls, hiding tired, puffy, wrinkled eyes under makeup, struggling into yet another "control" top that didn't, frustrated with my flab, upset with my weight, stressed out and angry at the diets that didn't work, the clothes that didn't fit, and the never-ending struggle with food that took over every waking moment of my life.

But there was more. In addition to just getting sick and tired of the extra weight I had been dragging around with me, like permanent luggage, for almost twenty years, I had begun to show signs of not feeling my best. I wasn't sleeping well. My sleep was often interrupted and then I couldn't go back to sleep for hours. I had become a real expert on television's predawn paid programming. Then there was this stiffness when I got up in the morning. I found myself shuffling off to the bathroom like someone twice my age. My mood wasn't so good either. I got into really down "blue" periods. I was tired all the time. And I was unbelievably cranky as though I had a permanent case of PMS . . . or worse, menopause! My skin showed fine lines and looked faded and tired. My pulse was high. So was my cholesterol and my blood pressure. I was getting older—and sicker, too.

THE END OF "YOUTH"

As the days of my "youth" drew to a close I decided to give it one more shot before it was too late.

I wasn't going to spend the rest of my life just sliding into middle age, then maturity and old age without making some attempt, once and for all, to have the body I always wanted.

And I did. I do. That was ten years ago! But back to my story.

Before I turned forty I lived with the hope, however unrealistic, that I would still have the figure I saw and envied in every women's magazine and on every commercial. I really believed I could still do it, that it wasn't too late. I believed I could lose the weight I struggled with all my life, get taut, have definition, look lithe, feel energized. I really believed that I could leave my bulging size sixteen (on a good day and on a lousy scale) behind and actually zip up—without having someone stand on my stomach—a size fourteen, then a size twelve, then a size ten, an eight, and even in my wildest fantasies (usually on the eve of yet another diet), a size six! Of course it was possible I kept reassuring myself, over and over again. I was young. I was healthy. All I needed was motivation. All I needed was to tap into that undiscovered source of willpower. All I needed was a miracle.

I would close my eyes and see my fantasy self slipping into a little black dress with spaghetti straps and not worrying about my upper arms shaking like some disgusting Jell-O mold. There she goes, the make-believe Edita, strolling casually down the street in tight white shorts not feeling two fat thighs rubbing together. I imagined myself pulling on a sweater, looking down and not seeing those two fleshy hills puffing up and over my bra like some four-breasted freak. But best of all, I pictured myself just throwing on a pair of jeans, leggings, a bathing suit, a skirt, a shirt, and not try to figure out yet another way to hide my fat.

ABANDON HOPE ALL YE WHO ENTER HERE

It wasn't that I hadn't tried to lose weight. Like thousands and thousands of other women I had tried every diet and every weight-loss program ever invented—twice—sometimes even three times. I was the perfect example of the triumph of hope over experience. Nothing worked.

And then the day I had been dreading for so long arrived. Here it was, my fortieth birthday. I had been a chubby teenager, a chunky young woman, and now I faced the grim prospect of being a dumpy, middle-aged matron. All my hopes of ever losing weight vanished. It was too late. I had missed the skinny ship. It was over. The sizzle left my life. So when I blew out the candles on my fortieth birthday cake (realize, I ate thirty-nine years of it myself in one sitting) I felt hopelessly fat, unattractive, and now, on top of everything else, old!

DOES OLDER MEAN FATTER?

Suddenly, everything was flat, like stale ginger ale, except for me. I was still round and destined to get even rounder. Because everyone knows that it's harder to lose weight the older you get. Right? And if I hadn't managed to drop an ounce when I was young—like yesterday—how could I possibly manage now that I had aged?

I began to get depressed. There were so many things I still wanted to do before it was too late. And the one thing I wanted to do more than anything else in the world was to lose weight. I couldn't kid myself anymore. Not only was I now middle-aged, but I was also fat. That's when panic and despair set in.

EDITA GETS HER FIRST GREAT IDEA AND CHANGES HER LIFE, BIG TIME!

What did I do? I did what any frustrated, depressed diet junkie would do. I went right to the fridge and while consoling myself with a pint of double fudge ice cream I decided to just stay fat. Simple. Dieting went out the window. In a way it was sort of a relief. It was as if I had given myself permission to finally stay fat. But while I came to somewhat reluctant and shaky terms with my weight, I wasn't ready to come to terms with my age. That's when I got my first great idea! Instead of focusing on losing pounds, I would focus on losing years. Believe me, at that point it seemed the easier of the two.

Little did I know that decision would change my life forever. Little did I know I would succeed in getting younger and as a wonderful, miraculous bonus, I would also finally lose the weight that defeated me my whole life. I threw my last coin into the fountain of youth and came up younger and thinner!

Let me tell you how this wonder of wonders came about.

As soon as I made the decision to push back the clock as far as I could, I did the obvious. I tried a new hairdo. I changed to softer makeup. I used lip liner to make bigger, younger lips. I thought cosmetic improvements would be enough. And they were, for a while. But my biological clock (not the one that starts ringing in baby time, but the one that chimes for every wrinkle and gray hair) was ticking and I was getting older by the minute. I still felt forty. And worse, I still looked forty. And what I wanted to avoid at all costs was feeling forty, and then feeling fifty and looking fifty—which I couldn't imagine but wasn't looking forward to.

WELCOME TO THE WONDERFUL WORLD OF LONGEVITY SCIENCE

In scouring all the women's magazines for tips on how to look younger I made a wonderful discovery. I found that there was a whole new body of science—longevity science—just in its infancy. I began to notice brief mentions of new research, new findings, new studies from respected scientific laboratories from around the world, all dedicated to understanding aging, slowing aging, and even reversing aging. I wasn't the only one it seemed who wanted to beat the clock. If aging could be slowed down, stopped, and even reversed from the inside out, it beat a new hairdo. And I was willing to live with the extra pounds if I could get some extra years.

I got hooked. My training as a medical journalist came in very handy at this stage. I found myself reading medical journals, textbooks, reports, and studies. I attended meetings and symposia. I interviewed experts in this new longevity science. And the more I researched and studied, the more excited I became. This was not some pie-in-the-sky stuff. This was happening right now, in my lifetime. Scientists, physicians, and researchers in a variety of fields were proving again and again that aging *can* be slowed, that aging *can* be reversed. The power to turn our biological clocks back was available to all of us. Why, I asked myself, wasn't this information out there? Why wasn't it "in my face"?

More questions bubbled up. How did all these scientists propose to make us younger? What was the plan? Was there a plan? When was the fountain of youth going to be built? When could I jump in? So what if I was going to jump in wearing a size eighteen bathing suit? Why did I have to go digging for nuggets of anti-aging findings in obscure, dusty journals? Why were the facts so hard to find? And why wasn't there a simple program that would allow me to put this research into immediate use?

THE SEARCH FOR MY FOUNTAIN OF YOUTH IS ON

And so I continued, faster and faster, deeper and deeper. I searched through the whole complex world of chemistry, physics, metaphysics, biology, anatomy, psychology, and physiology. I searched and searched. I read and reread. I wanted to find the formula. I wanted to make it easy. I wanted to slow down the ticking of my own aging clock. I wanted to get younger.

And then one day I found it. I couldn't believe it. There it was, the simple key to what all those scientists from all those disciplines were trying to tell us. The secret to getting younger was basic. It was as easy as breathing. I could hold it in my hand. I could start right away. And best of all I could eat it. It was in my very own fridge! Great, my favorite place!

AGING BY MOUTHFULS

I asked myself, what had I learned from all my research? I learned that scientists were pretty much agreed on one thing: We were making ourselves older, not with every passing day, but with every meal. We were speeding up our rate of disease. We were living longer, true, but we were spending those extra years in wheelchairs or attached to all kinds of machines that supported life but not living. We were living longer, but we were living fatter. We were digging our graves with a knife and fork at our own table. Conventional science had proven beyond a shadow of a doubt that what we eat makes us older and sicker. Now the new longevity science was proving that what we eat could make us healthier and younger!

It seemed so simple—too simple. And yet the proof was there. I had spent months and months looking for it. I had the research. I had the facts. I had put it together. Case after case of poor nutrition leading to heart disease, stroke, diabetes, cancer, osteoporosis, and all the other medical terrors that shorten our lives and make us old before our time. I didn't want my life shortened. I didn't want to get older faster, I wanted to get older slower . . . much, much, slower.

It made sense to me that if poor nutrition was the cause of premature aging, then good nutrition could give me back the stolen years and even add to them. Yes, of course it made sense. Wasn't that what all the publicity about cholesterol, saturated and unsaturated fat, excessive salt, and all the rest of the recent nutritional hoopla was about?

GETTING YOUNGER WITH EVERY BITE

Not quite. There was still something missing. And what was missing was the vital link between food and youth. It's one thing to eat to stay healthy; it's quite another to get younger with every bite. I still had a little more work to do. And I did it. It wasn't just any food that could make me younger. It wasn't just about calories, or fat, or cholesterol, or fiber. What should I do? Stop eating fat? Eat more fiber? Eat less salt? Give up white wine? Drink red wine? Go high protein? Go Mediterranean? If it was about food, then why didn't I, the ultimate diet junkie, look and feel younger already? What was missing? What was the secret? So what was the diet that could turn back the clock, that could make time march backwards, that could reduce my wrinkles, tighten my sags, give me the energy of a teenager, the complexion of a young woman, and the stamina of someone ten years younger than I was?

ANTI-AGING NUTRIENTS HAVE ARRIVED AND ARE ON YOUR GROCER'S SHELVES!

The answer was simple: antioxidants. Scientists had identified miraculous bundles of health and youth—anti-aging nutrients they named antioxidants—which were found only in very specific foods—not fancy foods, not expensive foods, not special foods, and not designer foods. Longevity scientists had discovered these anti-aging nutrients in common, everyday foods, that were in my own fridge, in my own supermarket!

HOW I ATE MYSELF OUT OF MIDDLE AGE

Great! The minute I figured this out I decided then and there to eat myself out of middle age. It sounded good. After all, eating was what I did best. Eating was what I loved. Terrific! Never mind about losing weight. I was going to lose years. I was finally going to stop worrying about getting thinner and concentrate on getting younger. I would stuff myself with "youth nutrients." And "stuff" was the key word. I knew myself well enough after a lifetime of on-again, off-again dieting to know that I would never be able to stay on any weight-loss program that measured food in skimpy ounces, tiny portions, and rigid three-meals-a-day regimens. So, if these youth nutrients were going to make up virtually my whole diet I wasn't going to skimp. I was going to gorge. The more I ate, I figured, the younger I would get.

EDITA GETS HER SECOND GREAT IDEA!

And that's when I got my second great idea. At first it seemed like I was really tempting fate. After all, wasn't it enough to get younger? I should be content with that discovery and concentrate on putting myself on an anti-aging diet. And yet I just couldn't shake the idea. It teased me. It tempted me. It haunted me. If certain nutrients—these antioxidants—could make me younger, I asked myself, could these same nutrients make me thinner? Was that too much to ask? Was I being piggy? No kidding?

Well, the answer to that question would change my life. Because ninety days later, not only was I more than ten years younger, but a fantastic twenty pounds thinner as well!

And so the *Fountain of Youth: The Anti-Aging Weight-Loss Program* was born!

HERE'S HOW I GOT MORE THAN TEN YEARS YOUNGER AND TWENTY POUNDS THINNER

First I spent months making endless lists and analyses of foods to determine which ones had the most anti-aging nutrients locked inside. Then I selected foods that were richest in anti-aging nutrients—antioxidants— and determined portions that would give me the anti-aging benefits of these youth nutrients. I also had to make sure that my total caloric intake would allow me to "stuff" myself and not pay the penalty in weight gain.

Once I settled on a ninety-day program of meals (which you will find faithfully reproduced for you to take your own voyage to youthfulness) I then had to determine exactly how old I was. I needed a starting point, something to refer back to as my Fountain of Youth program continued.

I knew how fat I was; I only had to step on my scale. Now I had to find out just how old I really was.

I got busy. Back to the research. And what did I find? I found, scattered in dozens of hard-to-find places, clues to testing true or actual age. And what exactly is true age? It isn't the date on the calendar. It isn't the number of candles on a birthday cake. It's biological age, the age of your body. And here's a shock: Your body could be three, five, ten, even fifteen years older than the calendar says it is.

The next part was both fun and scary. I put myself through a few simple tests that longevity scientists used to determine biological age. These tests were simple, easy, and fast. I did them in a few minutes. (You will have a chance to take these same tests in chapter 3.)

THE BIO-TESTS

I started in April. Here are the six tests I used to determine my own bio-age.

Bio-test #1 The Skin Pinch Bio-Test

April skin pinch test was 4 to 6 seconds.

This test was simple. All I had to do was lay my hand flat on a surface and take a pinch of skin from the top of my hand and keep pinching for five seconds. Then I had to let go and count how many seconds it took for the pinched skin to flatten out again. My result put my age at forty—close, since I was forty-one.

Bio-test #2 The Resting Heart Rate Bio-Test

April resting heart rate was 78 beats per minute.

Another piece of bad news. My resting heart rate showed my true age to be forty-nine—eight whole years older than I thought I was.

Bio-test #3 The Big Blur or Visual Acuity Bio-Test

April near vision was 10.8 to 11.3.

Near-vision blurring, or what I call the big blur test, is one of the key measurements of biological age. My score in this one put my age at forty-three—not great, but not too bad either.

Bio-test #4 The Systolic Blood Pressure Bio-Test

April blood pressure was 120/80.

Longevity scientists, focusing on the top number, the systolic pressure, put my age at thirty-seven. Great! So far, so good.

Bio-test #5 The Cholesterol Bio-Test

April cholesterol level was 220.

This was not so good. According to longevity tables, that reading put my age at forty-six—about five years biologically older than I really was.

Bio-test #6 The Weight Bio-Test

April weight was 168 pounds.

According to my scale I was fifty-five. This was a shock. I knew the scale was my enemy, but I didn't know until I weighed myself with my age in mind that I was fourteen years older than I thought.

Total Bio-Test Score

Then I added up all my age scores and divided that number by the number of tests. The result?

In April I was exactly forty-five years old. Not good, considering I was forty-one at the time.

I redid the tests just to make sure and the results were the same. I was forty-five years old—four years older than my calendar age. I breathed a sigh of relief. At least I wasn't ten years older.

ENTER MY FOUNTAIN OF YOUTH PROGRAM

Next I put myself on my own *Fountain of Youth* program. My goal? To stay on this program for ninety days and then do the tests over again. Remember, at this point all I wanted to do was to get biologically younger.

For ninety days I stuffed myself with foods rich in youth nutrients. All I wanted to do at that point was to prove that my chubby body could actually get younger with younger parts. I was going for the whole thing: younger skin, younger arteries, a younger heart, and even a younger brain.

I picked ninety days because many researchers felt that it took that long for the aging process to begin to reverse itself. It seemed fair to me. After all it had taken me forty-one years to become forty-five years old. I figured I could devote a mere ninety days to becoming, say forty or thirty-nine, or maybe if I were really lucky, thirty-five.

Well, you wouldn't believe what I ate. And how often. Suddenly I was eating not one skimpy meal a day, but six terrific and satisfying meals. I was eating all the time. Food tasted great! I was never hungry. I was spending less on groceries and enjoying my meals more than I ever had before. I was spending less time in the kitchen and the recipes I began to create looked good and tasted wonderful! I had no idea that antioxidants could be so good as well as so good for me.

IT'S WORKING . . . IT'S ACTUALLY WORKING!

And so the days went by. And I began to notice some pretty remarkable things. I wasn't tired all the time. I had loads of energy. My mood improved. I didn't get down or blue. My skin looked toned, faint lines faded, and my eyes got their sparkle back. The aches and pains I used to get disappeared as did the stiffness that had me stumbling and sore in the morning. My insomnia disappeared and I slipped easily and completely into wonderful, restful sleep. I stopped waking up halfway through the night, unable to get back to sleep without raiding the fridge. When morning came I was refreshed and eager for the day. Nothing bothered me. Little problems that used to frustrate me and leave me cranky and irritable were no longer overwhelming. I felt and looked and bounced around like someone ten years younger.

EVEN BETTER THAN I DREAMED

But it was my clothes that got me the most excited. They began to fit better. They were more comfortable. They didn't bind and pull the way they used to. My bras didn't dig and pinch and the elastic around my slacks didn't cut into my waist—I was even slowly developing a waist! I was actually losing weight. I was actually developing a shape that was different from my usual "round."

THE BIO-TESTS REVISITED AND
THE REMARKABLE RESULTS

And then the ninety days I had set for my program were over. And again, I put myself through the bio-tests I had taken a short three months before. Only this time the results were very different.

Check out these July results.

Bio-test #1 The Skin Pinch Bio-Test

I had improved my skin tone. Now instead of four to six seconds for it to get back to normal it took between two to four seconds. That reduced my biological age from forty in April to thirty in July.

Bio-test #2 The Resting Heart Rate Bio-Test

Back in April my resting heart rate had been seventy-eight beats per minute, which indicated a biological age of forty-nine. Now in July my resting heart rate had dropped to sixty-five beats per minute and put my age at twenty-five.

Bio-test #3 The Big Blur or Visual Acuity Bio-Test

Again, back in April my near vision had put me at forty-two. By July it hadn't really moved much. But I wasn't getting any older on this test anyway!

Bio-test #4 The Systolic Blood Pressure Bio-Test

My blood pressure dropped from 120/80 in April to 114/65 in July, making my biological age twenty-five.

Bio-test #5 The Cholesterol Bio-Test

My cholesterol dropped from 220 in April to 191 in July, reducing my biological age from forty-six to between thirty and thirty-nine. I picked thirty-nine in order to do the math.

Bio-test #6 The Weight Bio-Test

My weight had gone from 168 in April to 148 in July—a whopping twenty pounds. That reduced my age from fifty-five to a range between twenty-five and thirty-four. I picked thirty-four to do the math!

Total Bio-Test Score Ninety Days Later

I added up all the July scores, divided them by the number of tests, and couldn't believe my eyes. I had gone from a forty-one-year-old woman with a forty-five-year-old body to a forty-one-year-old woman with a thirty-two-and-a-half-year-old body! I had gotten twelve and a half years younger in just ninety days! And even better, I had lost twenty pounds, or almost 12 percent of my total body weight!

I had done it! I had found the Fountain of Youth. I had not only found it, but jumped right in with both feet! And I came up younger and thinner. And now you can too.

I WANT YOU TO KNOW WHY THIS IS A VERY SPECIAL BOOK

The *Fountain of Youth: The Anti-Aging Weight-Loss Program* gives you the tools to achieve a longer, healthier life and to lose weight in a healthy and satisfying way. These are the two most sought-after goals in our culture.

In fact youth and slenderness have been goals for centuries and across many cultures. Now, finally, that goal can be achieved for all of us. There is no deprivation. There are no expensive foods or formulas to buy. And there are no boring, frustrating diets to follow. Backed by the most current research in one of the most exciting fields of scientific study— longevity—*Fountain of Youth* integrates the theory of the laboratory with the practical application of the kitchen and dinner table.

Let's face it—we all want to live longer. We all want to be healthy. I can't think of a single person, including me, who isn't terrified at the thought of getting cancer, heart disease, having a stroke, falling down and breaking a bone, getting fragile and frail. None of us wants to spend the last twenty, thirty, or forty years of our lives trapped in wheelchairs or hospital beds. We want the same quality of life at sixty, seventy, or even ninety that we had at twenty. We want to feel and act as young as we think we are. I don't care if you are forty, fifty, sixty, or ninety, I'll bet deep down inside you still see yourself as much younger than the calendar indicates. I'll bet that in your own secret place you are sometimes shocked when you realize what your next birthday will be. Well, it doesn't have to shock you anymore.

GOOD NEWS FROM THE LONGEVITY FRONT

There is lots of good news on the longevity frontier. Today our average life expectancy is seventy-five and scientists believe that we can push the envelope even further in our own lifetime. In fact, a new study just released points out that women who have reached the age of fifty without any major diseases like cancer or heart disease have a good chance of living to ninety-two! And admit it, haven't you looked at some of those pictures in Willard Scott's gallery of 100 and 100-year-old-plus women (and men) and thought to yourself, *Wow, they look pretty good. I wonder if I'll make it to 100 and if I'll still be active and vital when I do?*

A QUICK LOOK AT SOME OF THE PROOF

Walter Bortz, M.D., in his book, *We Live Too Short and Die Too Long* (Bantam, 1991), observed, "Dr. Robert Butler, first director of the National Institute on Aging and long recognized as a master in the field of gerontology, has said, 'We haven't found any biologic reason *not* to live to 110.' I'll go a bit further. It is my best estimate that our biogenetic maximum life span is 120 years—approximately 1 million hours. This means that at birth we have the capacity to live that long."

And we now have the means, the information, the "stuff" to get there and still play a decent set of tennis doubles, take a walk, swim across a pool without drowning, or just enjoy our millionth sunset. Slowing, stopping, and even reversing the biological aging process is not some future "spacey" goal available to select rats in laboratories. No. The means to slowing, stopping, and even reversing biological age are available to all of us right now. We don't need any special training. There are no complex formulas to learn. It doesn't even cost much. And by slowing and reversing our own aging process, we can also finally, once and for all, lose those 5, 10, 50, or 100 pounds that have defeated us for years.

Saul Hendler, in his book *The Complete Guide to Anti-Aging Nutrients* (Fireside, 1984), asks, "We have among us a significant number of individuals who live into their eighties and nineties and even beyond with remarkable vigor and with relatively youthful appearance, individuals whose cardiovascular systems and mental faculties are, by objective standards and testing, the equal of those of healthy people in their thirties and forties. Why can't we all be like that or even better?" Then he goes on to answer his own question. "The answer is we can, using our current knowledge of nutrition . . . diet and nutrition are perhaps the most important factors . . . in the battle against premature aging."

The list goes on, folks.

Richard Earle, Ph.D., and David Imrie, M.D., of the Canadian Institute of Stress and authors of *Your Vitality Quotient* (Warner Books) state these current research findings:

- Many people *are* older than their years.
- You *can* reduce your biological age.
- You *can* look younger.
- You *can* feel better.
- People in their fifties or sixties *are able* to lower their body ages, as are people in their thirties or forties.

They went on to show in a remarkable study of over 600 subjects that within a few short weeks blood pressure decreased on average by 49 percent, cholesterol levels dropped by 50 percent, body fat decreased by 22 percent, and subjects became on average between two and one half and eight years younger, with some members of the study getting as much as twenty-five years younger!

So why doesn't this anti-aging message of hope get us all excited? Why aren't we turned on? Tuned in? Why aren't all of us jumping up and down with joy that we can live longer? Why? Because we are too busy being frustrated, confused, upset, and stressed out by the fact that we are fat and getting fatter. Because we face not only the problem of premature aging, but obesity as well. And we are not getting any thinner. The *New York Times* (March 8, 1994) reports, "Although they are eating less fat, Americans are consuming more rather than fewer calories, 231 more each day, to be exact."

And in light of this disturbing national trend the *Consumer Reports on Health* (September 1995) warns, "Overweight people who do nothing about their weight remain susceptible to a host of health problems: hypertension, high cholesterol, coronary disease, certain cancers, arthritis, gallstones, gout, low-back problems, and sleep disorders." The culprit is obesity.

These serious health problems shorten our lives. And this shortening of our life potential of 100-plus years is directly related to our excessive weight. It all comes down to the fact that we are eating ourselves into a premature old age.

But despite what expert after expert warns, quite frankly it is difficult, if not impossible, to deal with trying to get younger when so many of us haven't figured out how to get thinner yet. Well, now with the *Fountain of Youth: The Anti-Aging Weight-Loss Program* you can do both—get younger and thinner with every bite.

That's why *Fountain of Youth* is such a breakthrough book. It offers a practical, understandable program for not only reducing biological age but for reducing the weight that cuts off vital years through disease and premature death.

As a practical program, *Fountain of Youth* gives you the information you need to get your weight to a life-extending level.

Chapters are devoted to explaining in clear, simple language the revolutionary leaps in longevity research, the search for anti-aging nutrients hidden deep in our everyday foods, and the dissection of those foods to find the magic pellets called antioxidants that increase life span. There is a clear discussion of the major antioxidants—vitamin C, vitamin E, beta-carotene, and calcium—based on solid mainstream medical data, without resorting to the "fringy" and unfamiliar.

You will be given the tools to reduce age and weight in a safe, sensible way that fits into busy lives.

But the *Fountain of Youth: The Anti-Aging Weight-Loss Program* goes even further. It offers ninety days of planned foods, rich in anti-aging and weight-loss nutrients, to get you started on your new, slimmer, extended life. All you have to do is turn to each page and day after day eat yourself younger and slimmer with every bite. There are no meetings, no special foods to purchase, no complicated formulas to calculate, no bizarre ingredients to seek out in obscure specialty shops, and no expensive equipment to buy. *Fountain of Youth* shows you how to fit a youth and diet program into your life and the lives of your families with hardly a ripple to disturb the familiar patterns of eating and lifestyle.

According to *USA Today* (August 1995), America's favorite diet motivators are better health (67 percent) and improved appearance (21 percent)—both goals reachable through this program.

With only the chapters on longevity and obesity and their effects on your life combined with the ninety-day program of food selections, *Fountain of Youth: The Anti-Aging Weight-Loss Program* would be a breakthrough book. It more than satisfies the requirements set out by Deepak Chopra, M.D., in his book *Ageless Body, Timeless Mind* (Harmony, 1993), that a "healthy diet must have two components: (1) It has to be psychologically satisfying; (2) It has to provide a balanced supply of nutrients several times a day."

But *Fountain of Youth* goes even further. It doesn't leave you after ninety days. It holds your hand with an exciting cookbook offering 100 easy-to-fix, economical, and comforting recipes. There are breakfasts that give you a start on youth and weight loss even before you rush out the door in the morning. There are appetizers and snacks for the whole family that are good enough to serve at the most sophisticated party. There are wonderful salad combinations, soups, side dishes, main dishes for every season and mood; luscious desserts that look and taste sinful but are really "youth" concoctions; and there are healthy beverages to quench even the most picky thirst.

This is a trio of "must have" books all in one convenient place—your kitchen counter.

It is dedicated to giving you the two gifts that are precious beyond all things: a slender, healthy body and a way to turn back the aging clock of time.

Fountain of Youth works because:
- It is easy to follow.
- Results are fast.
- Results can be measured.
- There are no calories, fat grams, or anything else to count.
- Family and friends will notice the difference in your appearance.

- You'll enjoy eating again.
- You will reduce your risk of aging and life-shortening diseases.
- It is economical.
- You can do the program anywhere, anytime without feeling "out of it" at work, at home, at parties.

THE DEMOGRAPHICS OF PREMATURE AGING IN REVERSE

There could not be a better time for you to get with the *Fountain of Youth: The Anti-Aging Weight-Loss Program,* because according to the *New York Times* (September 1995), "The evidence continues to accumulate: for health and longevity, it pays to be thin. . . ."

Are you one of

- 75 million baby boomers
- 75 million mature Americans over fifty
- 100 million obese Americans?

There is growing support and interest in the media for all things dealing with diet and longevity.

Every newspaper, TV, and radio newscast focuses on the fat and age issues facing us today.

This book gives us all a lot of hope. We *can* do this. We *can* lose the weight. We *can* slow and even reverse our aging process. These issues continue to dominate the media. There is confusion, concern, and real fear as we reach each milestone birthday, whether it is forty, fifty, sixty, seventy, eighty, ninety, one hundred, or one hundred twenty. This book can help take away the fear of age, the frustration of weight, the confusion of how to stay healthy and active, and trade all those negatives for one big positive—more years to enjoy and live to the fullest—and slimmest.

Welcome to my Fountain of Youth!

PART ONE

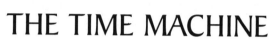

THE TIME MACHINE

CHAPTER 1

Longevity Science 101

What you are is God's gift to you.
What you become is your gift to God.

—ANONYMOUS

PETER PAN MEETS <u>THE BIG CHILL</u>

I first saw *Peter Pan* when I was a little girl with orange braids, freckles, and those cute Mary Jane socks with lace around the edges. I thought the dog was terrific. I loved the flying. And I wanted to grow up to be just like the ever-so-slightly-naughty Tinkerbell. If someone had asked me what the movie was about my answer was simple. To my seven-year-old mind it was about pirates, crocodiles, and running away from home.

Thirty years later, I saw *Peter Pan* again, this time with assorted nieces and nephews. They loved the dog. They loved the flying. And my favorite niece (bless her heart, may she grow up to be just like her Auntie Edita) wanted wings, stardust, the whole Tinkerbell number. What did they think it was about? Simple. They thought it was about pirates, crocodiles, and running away from home.

But this time, as I watched, I realized exactly what the movie was really about. It was about immortality. Forget Tinkerbell. This time around, I wanted to be Peter Pan. I wanted to be young and live forever.

THE FIRST SEXUAL REVOLUTION

You thought it was in the sixties, when Ozzie, Harriet, and Beaver turned into Elvis, Mick, and The Beatles. Wrong. The first sexual revolution was over fifty years ago when our parents (hard to believe, I know) grabbed each other, tumbled into the first available set of sheets, and didn't come up for air for two decades. That celebration of life produced a generation called baby boomers. That's us. From fifty-plus to thirtysomething we are 75 million strong and growing.

We're growing all right. We're growing older. We're growing fatter. We're growing sicker. That's the bad news.

We're also smarter, richer, and more powerful than any generation before us and possibly any generation that will follow. (Have you checked out Generation X lately?) We change things. We make things happen. And the next thing on our to-do list is to play *Beat the Clock* and win.

We don't want to be kids again. We don't want to be teens again. And we don't want to be twenty again. We just want to look and feel as though we were. We want to buy back the extra years as though we hadn't already spent them. We don't want to live forever—we just want to live longer. And we can.

WEIRD SCIENCE

We are not the first ones who wanted to slow down, stop, and even reverse the relentless and unforgiving march of time. Are you kidding? The search for the fountain of youth started the minute we were thrown out of the Garden of Eden and has progressed virtually uninterrupted from that moment to this.

Five thousand years ago a story was written down—it was the first story ever written. What was it about? A king who wanted to live forever. Gilgamesh was his name. And he went on a search for a magical plant that would make whoever ate it immortal. The plant, called the-old-men-are-young-again, grew under water. Gilgamesh was unsuccessful. He didn't find the plant or the secret of immortality. But that didn't stop thousands of years of searching for the fountain of youth—until now—when the baby boomers finally found it.

Consider.

Think anti-aging face creams are hot today? Check this out. The first ad for an anti-aging product appeared in an Egyptian newspaper called the Smith Papyrus in the year 2,900 B.C.! It advertised a paste that would smooth wrinkles and remove visible signs of aging. The whole thing came packaged in a fancy box inlaid with semiprecious stones. Nothing new there.

Then there was a do-it-yourself formula given to the legendary Jason of the Golden Fleece. It involved mixing together Oriental pebbles, moonlight frost, and wolf guts. Charming.

Then there was evidence left engraved on the tomb of an Egyptian who lived to be 115. His secret? The breath of young virgins.

Things got even weirder in the Middle Ages. Alchemists (pharmacists before chain drugstores) whipped up everything from potato milk shakes to cocktails made of babies' blood—all downed by their eager customers looking to fight back the visible signs of aging.

And then came the age of scientific discovery—and I use that term very loosely. Talk about your weird science. Enter a new gadget called the Vitalizer. It consisted of a flashlight, a metal rod, and a length of electrical cord. The idea was to insert the flashlight where the sun don't shine and plug into the nearest outlet. The youth boost was supposed to come from the electrical charge. (It's true. I can't make this stuff up, folks.)

Moving right along. In the mid-1950s a Romanian biochemist, Ana Aslan, claimed she found a drug, Gerovital-H3, which would cure aging. No matter that her miracle was mostly novocaine, the rush to her geriatric institute in Bucharest included Nikita Khrushchev and Charles de Gaulle and made the gold rush stampede look like a cake walk.

In Switzerland, even today, you can check into the famous Niehans Cellular Therapy Clinic. There, patients like Winston Churchill, Charlie Chaplin, and thousands more went (and still go) to get a syringe full of lamb fetus cells injected into their tushes to rejuvenate and retingle every little—and not so little—part of them.

The bottom line here is, we are not the first ones who wanted to stop and even reverse the march of time. We are, however, the first who have actually done it. Read on.

WHAT IS AGING ANYWAY?

According to two-time Nobel prizewinner Linus Pauling, "Aging is the process of growing old and approaching normal death. It is accompanied by a gradual deterioration in the biochemical and physiological functions."

We know what that means. It means:

- Graying, thinning hair
- Reading glasses, cataracts, and the big print edition of the newspaper
- Wrinkles, jowls, and liver spots
- Potbellies, flabby muscles, fallen arches, and an extra thirty pounds, mostly between our neck and knees
- Aching joints, broken bones, tennis elbow, hip replacements, and shrinking an inch
- Hot flashes, cold sweats, and sex hormones in little plastic bottles
- Indigestion, heartburn, and never being more than thirty seconds from the nearest bathroom
- Skin cancer, breast cancer, colon cancer, lung cancer, and every other major cancer around
- Head colds, chest colds, flu shots, and pneumonia
- Forgetting the keys, forgetting the car, forgetting the kids
- Clogged arteries, high blood pressure, strokes, and cardiac arrest
- Hearing aids, walkers, and adult diapers

And that's just the stuff you can see for yourself. Meantime, on the cellular level, other changes due to age are taking place.

A SNEAK PEEK AT YOUR AGING BODY

Brain weight	Decreases 40%
Blood flow to the brain	Decreases 20%
Kidney filtration rate	Decreases 50%
Metabolic rate	Decreases 20%
Lung volume during exercise	Decreases 47%
Resting heart output	Decreases 30%
Handgrip strength	Decreases 45%
Oxygen uptake while exercising	Decreases 60%
Total muscle	Decreases 20%
Aerobic capacity	Decreases 40%

Blood pressure and cholesterol levels go up.
Ratio of body fat to muscle doubles.
Body temperature goes down.

Not a very cheerful prospect. And all this aging starts rushing at us sometime shortly after our thirtieth birthday. That's why we really don't need fancy scientific definitions of aging. We know what aging is. It doesn't take a genius. All it takes is a mirror. We also know about the speed of aging. Every year past thirty feels like we are aging faster and faster, racing to the inevitable end, like some demented ride in a real-life twilight zone. What we want to know is how to stop it, slow it down, reverse it. That's what we want to know about aging.

SO, HOW LONG HAVE WE GOT?

One million hours, or 120 years, say the experts. So, if you are reading this and you are thirty-five you potentially have another eighty-five years to go. If you are forty you've got another two entire lifetimes ahead of you. And if you are fifty, sixty, or seventy, you've got enough time to graduate from college more than ten times over.

> We have the potential to live six times as long as it took our bones to fully form. The adult skeleton is fully developed at age twenty. Multiply 20 times 6 and you have 120, or 1 million hours.
>
> —GEORGE BUFFON, French biologist

That's the potential. That's our life span. Now here is the reality. This is our life expectancy.

REALITY CHECK
LIFE EXPECTANCY IN OUR TIME

How to read this chart: Find your age range in the first column. Then go across to your life expectancy in either the men's or women's column on the right. That's what's left.

Age Range	Average Years of Life Remaining for a Male in This Age Range	Average Years of Life Remaining for a Female in This Age Range
0–1	71.8	78.6
1–5	71.6	78.3
5–10	67.8	74.4
10–15	62.8	69.5
15–20	57.9	64.6
20–25	53.3	59.7
25–30	48.7	54.9
30–35	44.1	50.1
35–40	39.6	45.3
40–45	35.1	40.5
45–50	30.7	35.8
50–55	26.4	31.3
55–60	22.3	26.9
60–65	18.6	22.7
65–70	15.2	18.8
70–75	12.1	15.2
75–80	9.4	11.9
80–85	7.1	9.0
85 plus	5.3	6.6

Source: National Center for Health Statistics

Life span = 120 years
Life expectancy = 75 years

CLOSE, BUT NO CIGAR

So, you've noticed. Although we have the potential to live to 120 years, the reality is unpleasantly different. We are getting closer, we're just not there yet. On the other hand, just look how far we've come.

In a Japanese burial ground 236 skeletons were found that were estimated to be seven thousand years old. Scientists were able to determine that the average body buried there never made it past fifteen.

There is a cemetery on the island of Cyprus that researchers believe is over five thousand years old. Tests on those bodies buried there show life expectancy at birth way back then was sixteen.

In the Stone Age life expectancy was seventeen.

Even though ancient Greeks influenced our thinking for almost three thousand years, they couldn't extend their own lives much past the age of thirty.

The same goes for the mighty Romans. An examination of Roman epitaphs on over ten thousand gravestones found that the average age at death was twenty-two.

At the time of the American Revolution, the average age at death for most colonists in this brave new world was thirty-five.

By the turn of this century, 1900, things were better and Americans were living to the ripe old age of forty-seven!

Ninety-plus years later, we have extended our lives, finally reaching that biblical "three score years and ten" and even beating it by a few years or so, to seventy-five. That's a jump of almost thirty years in just one century! We're getting closer, but we still have a long way to go.

Explorer Juan Ponce de Leon was 53 when he set out to look for the fountain of youth in 1513. By the life expectancy standards of the Middle Ages, that made him a very old man, indeed.

So what's the forecast? Are we going to be able to live those 1 million hours? Are we going to make it to 120? Some of us will. But not very many. By the year 2050 the average life expectancy will be 100 (103 for women). How many of us will reach that magic number? Again experts agree. There will be 1 million Americans over the age of 100. The question is, will one of them be you?

SO MUCH FOR THE "WEAKER" SEX

One thing is for sure, most of those 1 million 100-year-olds are going to be women. Numbers don't lie. Women are no longer the weaker sex. Au contraire. Men are dropping like fruit flies and women are just going on and on and on like that pink and fuzzy Energizer bunny. Why is that?

For most of history women have had an equal or shorter life expectancy than men. Why? Kids, that's why. Kids could—and did—kill you. Having them was life threatening (the more things change the more they stay the same—isn't that the truth?). But over centuries of evolution women adapted. We got tougher, stronger, more resilient. We had to. Did you think cavemen were actually going to stay in the cave all day and raise the kids? Not a chance. Over time, nature gave women a slight edge.

The rest was your basic clean hands. Once doctors started to wash their hands, more and more women survived actual childbirth without the risk of postnatal infection.

Today the rate of death for women remains close to one-half that for men. Studies show women start life in better shape than their baby brothers and by age thirty-five are twice as healthy as their spouses. We begin to lose some of that advantage as we get older. So let's not pat ourselves on the back just yet, ladies, and let's not celebrate our potential longevity with another cookie—or three.

WE'VE WON A FEW BATTLES—BUT THE WAR "AIN'T" OVER

We have won a few major battles against age and have gotten a little closer to that magic 120 years. But for the vast majority of us, men and women alike, our human potential might as well be science fiction. We aren't going to make it to 120. Most of us aren't going to make it to 100 or even 80. And those of us who do are probably going to spend at least twenty or more years in pain, gradually getting more and more worn-out, sicker and sicker, confined to walkers, then wheelchairs, and finally nursing homes. That's our reality.

We have improved medicine, conquered most infectious diseases, dis-

covered hygiene, spent fortunes on health care, and amassed an unprece-
dented amount of information about living to the max. So why aren't we?
Why aren't we living to the max? Why will only 1 million of us make it
to 100? Why will even fewer of us make it to 120? What's the problem?
Why is life still a fatal disease?

THE TOP TEN HIT PARADE OF PROVEN LIFE SPANS

Animal	Years
Tortoise	150
Man	113
Elephant	60
Orangutan	58
Gorilla	55
Chimpanzee	50
Eagle	50
Whale	50
Horse	40
Grizzly bear	35

SOLVING THE RIDDLE OF WHY WE AGE

It isn't enough to know *how* we age, we need to understand *why* we age
in the first place. We need to understand why some of us age faster than
others. We need to understand why some of us get wrinkles at forty and
others have smooth skin at sixty, why some of us break a hip at fifty-five
while others are out playing tennis at seventy, why some of us will get
cancer, strokes, heart disease, diabetes, Alzheimer's, and all the other diseases of aging and others won't.

Scientists believe that if the riddle of why we age can be solved, aging
and the diseases it brings can be slowed, stopped, and even cured. And
many of those same scientists believe that the riddle of age has already
been solved. They believe that our own bodies have slowly unlocked the
secret of long life stored in every single one of our 50 trillion cells. They
believe the fountain of youth is available to all of us right now. We can
turn back our own aging clocks. We can go backwards in time to when
our bodies were five, ten, fifteen, even twenty years younger. And we can
look forward to living healthy active lives. They believe that every one of

us can live to a vigorous and happy 85, 95, and even 120. I believe it too. And when you have read this book and completed this program, you will believe it also. Why? Because you will be able to turn back your own aging clock and be younger than you are today.

LOOK WHO'S FIFTY AND COUNTING

Oliver Stone	Dolly Parton
Joe Greene	Gene Siskel
Susan Sarandon	Gregory Hines
Suzanne Somers	Candice Bergen
Pat Sajak	Reggie Jackson
Diane Keaton	Cher

THE THEORIES OF AGING

There are many theories why we age and why so few of us reach our full calendar potential. Most of these theories fall into two main categories: damage theories and preprogrammed theories.

Damage theories are based on the premise that our life essence gets worn out, rusted, and falls apart like an old car or outdated appliance.

The preprogrammed theories, on the other hand, tell us that we are stuck with a future we can't control. Our life timer has been set. That timer determines the length of our childhood, triggers those teen hormones, determines the year of our menopause, and is going to go off when we do.

But whatever the theory, with the addition of new scientific findings, with the unrelenting quest by some of the most brilliant minds in the world, the why of aging has now come clearer. And the answer may lie in a most unlikely place. You'll see.

The Rate of Living Theory

By the turn of this century, the first tentative experiments to understand human aging were under way. A researcher at Johns Hopkins University proposed a theory that the longevity of animals was the direct expression of metabolic rate. What he was saying was, the faster our bodies run, the faster they wear out. He called this the rate of living theory. He postulated that one way to live longer is to slow down our metabolic and chemical rates. How? By cooling them. Think about it. At the North Pole icebergs last forever. At the equator, they turn into water and disappear.

Good theory, but there are a couple of flaws. If frozen things lasted longer, why didn't Eskimos live longer than sun bunnies?

Don't move to that retirement community north of Alaska just yet. Don't give up those golf clubs for ice fishing equipment just yet. The search went on.

The Carrel Immortality Theory

In 1912 at the Rockefeller Institute Dr. Alexis Carrel, a Nobel prizewinning biologist and the "grandfather" of longevity science, put a bunch of human cells called fibroblasts (the building blocks of collagen) into bottles. He fed these experimental cells a special blend of cell food. They divided really well. He kept feeding them and they kept right on dividing for thirty-four years! In fact, they ultimately outlived him.

What did he conclude from his experiment? Carrel believed that human cells, given the right environment, are immortal. Cells die, he decided, because something messes up their perfect environment.

This was the prevailing theory for about fifty years. And then it was totally and completely shattered.

The Hayflick Limit Theory

This is the primal theory. This is the theory that brought aging out of the superstitious and often ridiculous world of goat testicles and wings of blue and white butterflies caught by the light of the moon on the second Tuesday of months that end in r. This is the theory that brought the fight against aging into the modern world of cellular research and launched the field of longevity science.

In the mid-1960s gerontologist Leonard Hayflick decided to reproduce Carrel's experiment and see for himself whether or not human cells were really immortal. So he followed the recipe. He put a bunch of normal human cells, fibroblasts, in a petri dish. He fed them like Carrel had. He watched them. Hayflick's fibroblast cells divided like all good and healthy cells do, and divided again, and once again. They divided a total of fifty times. And then they stopped dividing and died.

Hayflick noticed something else. He noticed that the closer the cells got to the fiftieth division the slower they divided. Next he tried adding a variable. He took a bunch of cells that had divided about thirty times already and froze them. The idea was to trick them into thinking that they were starting their cellular division from square one when they were thawed out. Sounded like a good idea, except once they were unfrozen, Hayflick's cells "remembered" that they had already divided thirty times before they were frozen and so merrily divided exactly twenty more times.

There it was. Fresh or frozen, it made no difference. Cells divided a set number of times, slowed down, and died. If the cells were in a warm room, they divided faster, but they still divided fifty times. If they were in a cold room they doubled slower, but the number fifty was fixed. When Hayflick put the cells of older people into his little lab jars they doubled fewer times than cells of much younger volunteers.

What did Hayflick conclude? His first conclusion was that his buddy Carrel must have somehow accidentally kept adding fresh cells to his cell soup when he added fresh food to their environment. Given the state of instruments back then, that was probably exactly what had happened.

But Hayflick did something that no other researchers into the mysteries of human aging had been able to do. He found the human cellular clock. He proved human cells are preprogrammed to die after they have reproduced themselves fifty times. And that program is locked into each cell with a genetic password. We can't crack the code. So said Hayflick.

Sounds kind of hopeless, right? It would be except for a couple of very interesting deviations from this theory of aging. There are cells that don't die, immortal cells, cells that keep on doubling, and doubling, and doubling forever. These cells have somehow turned off the molecular alarm clock that signals the end of living and the beginning of dying. Unfortunately these eternal cells are cancer cells. Hayflick found the clock. The question then became how to turn on that death signal to cancer cells and turn it off to normal healthy cells.

The second question raised by the Hayflick theory is how come some of us live longer than others. If we are all programmed to drop dead after our cells divide about fifty times, why do some of us live to only 45 while others live to 95 and why do so few of us live to 120?

The answer, some scientists believe, may lie in the fact that we do things to speed up our own cell divisions. We are accelerating our own rate of aging. Read on and find out how to take your foot off the accelerator of aging and put it on the brake.

The Wear and Tear Theory

This popular theory likens us to a late-model car. Filled with the right gas, oil changed regularly, spark plugs cleaned, and driven only to church on Sundays in southern Florida, this vehicle is going to last for years. Now take that same car and drive it into the ground, leave it out in the snow, let winter salt corrode its underbelly, ignore every little red warning light, and pump in whatever gas is cheapest and that car is going to die on you in the middle of some interstate real soon.

The same idea is presented about us. We just wear out and rust out like some old car sitting in the front yard on blocks with dusty weeds growing out of its busted windows.

This is an easy theory to believe. When we look into a mirror some of us see a kind of human wreck: bags and wrinkles, age spots, hunched-over shoulders, stiff joints, worn out and rusted out, just like some old car.

Well, what's wrong with this theory? Plenty. First of all, we aren't a car. Second of all, it still doesn't explain why we age at different rates and die at different rates and why more of us don't become 120-year-old vintage classics.

So the search for why we age continues.

The Chaos Theory

This one is kind of cosmic. It says that aging is the effect of energy on matter over time. The longer we live, the more we get bashed about by the "slings and arrows of outrageous fortune" and when we've been bashed to the max, all the energy that kept our bits and pieces of cells together in the shape of a human lets go and we sort of disintegrate and succumb to the natural law of decay.

Some of us, the proponents of this theory argue, have more energy to begin with and so can hold their shape better and last longer.

The Crosslink Theory

If you've ever heard the expression "a stiff," meaning a corpse, you will understand the crosslink theory. This theory, first expressed by Johan Bjorksten, states that migrant molecules that penetrate our cells join up with each other and "gum up" the inner works. Some of these molecules are a kind of cellular garbage we throw off as a result of breathing, eating, walking, sleeping, and everything else. These bunches of sticky molecules attach themselves like a spider web across our joints and muscles. The longer we live, the more of these webs build up. The first sign we may have that we have been invaded by crosslinking molecules is morning stiffness. Start shuffling off to the bathroom or down the stairs and those little sticky molecules have you in their grip. Most of us can deal with the morning stiffness, but it doesn't stop there. That sticky web is spreading all over our connective tissues, getting closer and closer to our DNA— the master program for each one of our cells. Finally, cell after cell succumbs and stiffens. And then we die.

Again, some of us never stiffen up. And some can't even lift a golf club after the age of fifty. Can we melt the glue that is gumming up our works? Keep reading.

The Death Gene Theory

A recent headline in the *New York Times* read "Scientists Discover Gene Affecting Aging" based on a study reported in a highly respected journal, *Science*. As with all discoveries, this one raises more questions than it answers. The initial study was conducted on people suffering from a fairly rare inherited disorder called Werner's syndrome. This disorder speeds up human aging so that teenagers develop wrinkles, gray hair, cataracts, and osteoporosis. By the time they are in their twenties victims of Werner's syndrome have heart disease, high blood pressure, and cancer. They die with the bodies of eighty-year-olds in their thirties or early forties. Scientists, it was reported, found the gene sitting on the top of chromosome number eight that may be responsible for this disease and may also regulate the speed of human aging.

Does this mean that for some of us this gene is damaged and we age faster? Can we do anything to "fix" the gene? And how important is it, really, in normal human aging?

The Specific Metabolic Rate Theory

This can also be called the "first you eat, then you die" theory. It goes like this. Did you know that nearly all animals use up the same amount of chemical energy in their lifetimes? Scientists have figured it out to be about 25 to 40 million calories per pound per lifetime. So a mouse will burn the same number of calories per pound in a lifetime of three years as an elephant burns in his sixty years. We are the lucky exception to this rule. We get to consume about 80 million calories per pound before we've taken our last bite and the system shuts down. Now, do you still feel like that 2,000-calorie slice of chocolate cake or do you want to rethink your next snack?

The Free Radical Theory

And the winner is the free radical theory of aging! After all the other theories, speculations, and experiments this is now the prevailing theory of why we age. And it is this theory that not only explains the aging process, but offers us some very exciting and achievable ways to fight back and win.

This theory, which today is number one on the anti-aging hit parade, will take a little getting used to because it tells us something that turns one of our fundamental beliefs about the physical universe we live in completely topsy-turvy.

First, let's meet some of these free radicals. They know you very well; it's time you got to know them. Free radicals have been around for a long time in chemistry. In fact, without free radicals we wouldn't have plastic wrap, plastic bottles, plastic garbage bags, plastic toys—we wouldn't have plastic.

Scientifically, they are part of the stag line at the cellular prom. Free radicals are like a bunch of guys who have come to the dance without a date. And so they kind of roam around the edges, have a drink or two for courage, and then zap—one of them pounces on a cute sophomore whose real date has gone to the loo for a minute. The nasty free radical whisks her away for a dance. Meantime, her date comes back, tries to cut in on the intruder, and before you know it, there is pushing and shoving, noses get broken, fists fly, the band stops playing, other guys get involved (it's kind of a guy thing), and pretty soon the place is trashed. The sweet young couple go home, bruised, shaken, and damaged. And what about the free radical and his friends? They move on to another cellular dance and the whole scene is repeated again and again.

Free radicals have been called the "great white sharks" of our very life essence. Free radicals were first identified as human life force scavengers by Dr. Denham Harman of the University of Nebraska. To him goes the credit for developing the free radical theory of aging in the mid-1950s in which he suggested that free radicals were the primary cause of aging at the cellular level.

So what are they? This is where our preconceived notions get challenged, folks. Think of yourself as now entering a molecular parallel universe. Free radicals are the dark side of oxygen. That's right. The very stuff that we need to live, oxygen, is also in some weird and totally unfunny cosmic joke killing us with every breath. Free radicals are oxygen atoms that have an extra electrical charge or extra electron. This makes them wobbly and unstable. So they run around our cellular substructure looking to latch onto another electron for stability (just like that single guy at the prom with too much to drink). In the process of rushing around they damage delicate cell walls, causing vital fluids to leak out. They rape other molecules looking for a stabilizing electron. They intercept DNA transmissions and garble important genetic messages. Suddenly cells get the wrong message and start reproducing in strange ways, altering the genetic blueprint and creating mutants, the precursors of disease. Free radicals are big trouble.

If you don't believe this, just look at a piece of apple cut up and left on the counter. See the brown? That's what free radicals do to stuff that is exposed to oxygen. Remember that garden furniture you didn't paint? Remember the rust? That's what free radicals do to metal exposed to oxygen. And what about that pound of butter you forgot to put away? Rancid, right? Free radicals and oxygen again. Now look in the mirror. See those wrinkles? See those darkish aging spots? That's right. Free radicals and oxygen and you. Now can you imagine what is going on inside you at the cellular level, at the microscopic level, at the aging level itself when free radicals are let loose? Free radicals speed the formation of heart attack-causing cholesterol, they stimulate the formation and growth of cancer cells, they destroy the message centers in the brain and speed the onset of Alzheimer's. They are nasty and they cause us to age and sicken well before our time. In countless studies free radicals have been shown to be responsible for some of the worst killer diseases we are still battling. They upset the delicate balance that keeps us well and alive.

How did they get into our cells in the first place? Well, here's where you really have to take a scientific leap of faith. We breathe them in with every breath of oxygen we take, with every breath of oxygen we need to live. We also produce them every time we digest a meal, every time our heart beats, every time we do a math problem. Free radicals are the result of normal functioning. They are by-products, the waste of living. Free radicals are part of the whole package of life and age and death, and there's not much we can do about that.

But that's not the only way these cellular rapists got in. If it was only through breathing, or eating, or thinking, our normal defense systems would probably do the job and disarm them and we might not have to worry about free radical damage. But we are the agents of excessive free radical damage. We are the ones who help overload our own bodies' defense systems. We are the all too often willing accomplices in our own cellular destruction. We open the doors wide to free radical scavengers and damage with every cigarette we smoke or every puff of polluted air we swallow. We get them started with every slice of processed meat like bacon and sausage we cook up. We give them free rein to do their damage by eating extra fat, by living stressful lives. They love a drink or three. (I think vodka is their favorite.) We invite them in every time we expose ourselves to the sun directly without any sunscreen protection.

It is estimated that our bodies suffer 10,000 free radical "hits" every day.

So what do we know? We know that free radicals are the damage makers, the age makers. They are invisible to the naked eye but the damage they do can shorten our lives by vital years. They can force us into wheelchairs. They can scramble our brains. They can wrinkle our skin, weaken our eyesight and hearing, and stop our hearts. Free radicals make us old before our time and then in the end they can kill us.

Is there anything that can stop free radicals from doing serious damage? You bet. Cellular cops, called antioxidants. Antioxidants are like a free radical swat team—an elite force of free radical destroyers headed up by Sylvester Stallone, Arnold Schwarzenegger, and Clint Eastwood, and they are what the rest of this book is all about.

CHAPTER 2

The Unholy Trinity:
Fat, Food, and Age

Fat people die young.

—HIPPOCRATES

THE GREAT AMERICAN PIG-OUT

Well, we've finally done it. That is, at least 80 percent of us have done it. We're living in hog heaven. That's right. We've moved in and brought our friends, our spouses, and even our kids along. Used to be kind of a quiet neighborhood, but not anymore. Hog heaven is getting mighty crowded these days.

THE FAT STATS

There is a ten-year game plan set out by the surgeon general called Healthy People 2000. The goal was to have a nation of healthy, slender Americans all toasting in a new century with bubbly carrot juice cocktails. Well, it doesn't look like it's going to happen. In fact, we are going backwards. More toward the Unhealthy People 2000. Instead of lean, mean fighting machines, more and more of us are soft, mushy fatsos—64 percent of all of us—that's 98 million from sea to shining sea. (Some studies show fewer chubbies, some show more, but the bottom line is our bottoms are widening as well as our tops.) How many is 98 million? Well, it's pretty much everybody in New York and California and most places in between. (I think there may be some lean and healthy people in Montana and I know there's a couple more in South Dakota, but they are going to get sucked in soon.) In fact, some are even predicting that by the new century every adult in America will be overweight.

The percentage of overweight Americans was 8 percent more
in 1995 than in 1985.
Guess who's winning the fat contest?
Women.

Not a day goes by without some new study or other warning us about the danger of being overweight or obese. Even gaining as few as eleven pounds puts us at a much greater risk for life-shortening diseases. One-third of all cancer deaths and more than one-half of all cardiovascular deaths are the direct result of overweight. But we don't hear any of these lifesaving warnings. Why? Because the sound of crunching potato chips is drowning out the messages.

The mean body weight of Americans has increased by 7.9 pounds
over the past fifteen years and is still rising.

This is no longer funny. Fat lady jokes aren't. This is no longer vain or trivial. This goes way beyond wanting to zip up last year's dress for this year's party. This goes way beyond an hour of embarrassment at some weekly weight-loss meeting or a $300 investment in prepackaged diet food.

Even though some studies show that we are slowly getting the fat out of our diets, we are replacing it with extra calories, exactly 231 extra calories every single day. The result? We're still getting fatter. This is serious. This is scary.

We are dying here. Between the grocery store and our own kitchen table, we are committing nutritional suicide. There isn't a family in America who isn't affected by the killer results of fat. Our mothers get strokes. Our fathers have heart attacks. Our kids have high cholesterol. Our spouses have hypertension. And we are walking cancer factories. And what's our biggest concern? Finding our waistline before next Friday night.

And do you know what the real tragedy is here? In labs all over this country—all over the world—scientists are working to unlock those final few secrets of longer life. Miracles in longevity are happening. We are the first generation in the entire history of recorded time that can live to be 120 years old. There it is. The maximum life span achieved. What a mountain to have climbed! What a peak to have scaled! And do you know what? Most of us can't even make it up one single flight of stairs!

> The average weight of men in their forties is 173 pounds compared with 140 pounds 100 years ago.
> The average weight of women in their forties is 140 pounds compared with 128 pounds one hundred years ago.

MIRROR, MIRROR ON THE WALL, WHO IS THE FATTEST OF THEM ALL?

If it were only about fat, this would be just another low-fat book. But there's more to it than that. It's about making the right food decisions. It's about knowing what foods will fight off cancer, heart disease, stroke, hypertension, osteoporosis, diabetes, depression, and aging. It's about grasping the fact that there is only so much room in each food for various elements. Some of those elements are vitamins. Some are minerals. Some are protein. And some are fat. It's understanding that the more fat there is in a particular food, the less room there is for other elements, just like in us. The more fat there is in us, the less room there is for all those nutrients that extend our youth and our lives.

> The American Dietetic Association says more than 82 percent of Americans recognize the importance of good nutrition, but only 39 percent (down from previous years) say they are doing all they can to achieve a healthy diet.

Test Your Fountain of Youth Nutritional Savvy

You have a pretty good concept of what is good for you and your family and what isn't, so you think. And anyway, it's just all too complicated: too many choices, too much conflicting food news, too little time to cook from scratch, too confusing to read labels, too much of a hassle to fight over nutrition with family. Have I missed any excuse? Have I left out any reason for not getting smart about what we eat and what we don't? Let's see just how really smart we are about nutrition. Let's see how well we take care of ourselves and the families we love. Come on, let's take this little nutrition IQ test.

1. No time to fix breakfast. What's a better bet, a bagel with some cream cheese or a bran muffin when you're on the run?
   A bagel with cream cheese has only 300 calories and 11 grams of fat compared to a six-ounce average bran muffin, which has 600 calories and a disgusting 22 grams of fat.
2. It's movie time. The best choice for a movie snack is a small tub of unbuttered popcorn, a box of chocolate-covered raisins, or a package of red licorice sticks.
   Pick the licorice. It is practically fat free and half a package is about 260 calories. Compared to 10 grams of fat in raisins or unbuttered popcorn, your choice is clear.
3. You get the most calcium from milk, broccoli, spinach, or kale?
   A new study has found that we absorb more calcium from kale than from milk, broccoli, or spinach.
4. Which is more nutritious, cooked carrots or raw carrots?
   This is one time where cooked, as in lightly steamed, releases more beta-carotene, an important antioxidant, than raw.
5. Which is most heart-smart, white wine or purple grape juice?
   Wine has gotten all the press, but purple grape juice contains the

same heart-saving substance from the skin of grapes that red wine does. Also, wine tends to make people eat more. So purple grape juice is a better pick.

6. What has more calories, a baked potato with cheese sauce or an order of French fries?

    If you really have to, go for the fries. A baked potato with cheese weighs in at 475 calories and 29 grams of fat. Fries come in at 234 calories and 12 grams of fat. But your best bet is still the baked potato without the cheese.

7. Which of these so-called goodies has the most fat, a double burger with the works, ½ cup of premium ice cream, a fast-food salad with a packet of ranch dressing, or a fast-food order of large fries?

    The salad with the dressing. Surprised? Shocked? A packet of ranch salad dressing adds 30 grams of fat—about half or more of your daily allowance—and wipes out any virtue of picking the salad in the first place. You were good to pick the salad; next time bring your own nonfat dressing with you and you'll be a winner.

8. Which deli sandwich is usually the lowest in fat and makes the best choice for an office lunch—ham, chicken salad, tuna salad, or sliced turkey?

    Sliced turkey is the best bet. Ham is fatty and chicken and tuna salads are usually made with mayo. So go for sliced turkey or chicken with a little mustard and lettuce and tomato for a good lunch.

9. How many servings of fruits and veggies are we supposed to eat every day to get the minimum amount of anti-aging vitamins? Is it three, five, eight, ten, or fifteen?

    The minimum is five a day. But we should all really be getting at least ten for optimum anti-aging benefits. What's a serving? About ½ cup. Even veggie haters should be able to manage that.

10. What are the most important anti-aging weight-loss nutrients we need every day?

    The answer is vitamin C, vitamin E, beta-carotene, and calcium. And if you didn't know that, keep reading—it could save your life and buy you an extra five, ten, or more years.

Well, how did you do? How well do you really know what you are feeding your face, your skin, your arteries, your brain, and every single one of your rapidly aging chubby cells? If you got even one answer wrong on the nutrition quiz you are in danger of making wrong food choices every single day. And each wrong choice compounds itself day after day until you have fewer and fewer days left.

But making those choices is getting tougher all the time. Who would have figured that a bagel with cream cheese was better than a bran muffin? Oh, sure, we all know the bagel is fine. But the messages about cream cheese have us saving it for a special Sunday brunch, while we go ahead and scarf down a couple of bran muffins. And you know what, bran muffins aren't even that good. They taste like, well, like bran.

And what about that baked potato versus French fries? I bet we all thought that melted cheese was a great idea—lots of calcium there—so we wolf down tons of extra fat thinking we're getting thin.

And then the real shocker. The salad. Oh, sure, we all know that salad dressing is not the best choice, but how is it possible that one of those little bitty plastic pouches that you can hardly open most of the time can sabotage our entire food day so badly.

No wonder we are getting fatter. No wonder we are getting sicker. No wonder we are getting older. It's a nutritional minefield out there and too many of us are getting blown up.

It gets worse. Not only have most of us completely lost it when it comes to something as basic as our food, but those researchers out there keep shifting the fat floor from beneath our feet.

The Bathroom Scale Revisited

Who says scientists are perfect? Sometimes even the best of them make mistakes. And the bathroom scale was one. Back in 1959 while Elvis was shimmying and shaking, the Metropolitan Life Insurance Company published a chart of ideal weights based on actuarial probabilities. In 1990, the United States Departments of Agriculture and Health and Human Services published a table of weight guidelines. The 1990 chart was a lot more generous and allowed added pounds with added years. Great, many of us thought. We weren't as overweight as we had thought. We were going to be fine. Those few extra pounds were normal, natural, healthy. Getting a little heavier as we got older wasn't going to kill us—the government said so. What a relief we felt when we unbuckled our belts that extra notch and lost the guilt.

Now experts are in the middle of a scientific version of a food fight over which of these tables is best. Some experts believe that it is fine for us to gain a little weight as we get older. Others think that's the worse possible scenario and poses a real threat to our longevity. The fact that we are getting fatter and sicker younger sort of has me thinking that maybe those folks back in the 1950s were right. Since most of us are seriously fat and dying prematurely it seems that less is more. Get on your scale and see for yourself.

WEIGHT TABLES 1959 VS. 1990

CIRCA 1959

This table is based on a chart published by the Metropolitan Life Insurance Company in 1959. This austere guide is as stringent for the teenager as it is for the retiree.

HEIGHT	WEIGHT (LBS.) Women	Men
5'0"	103–115	—
5'1"	106–118	111–122
5'2"	109–122	114–126
5'3"	112–126	117–129
5'4"	116–131	120–132
5'5"	120–135	123–136
5'6"	124–139	127–140
5'7"	128–143	131–145
5'8"	132–147	135–149
5'9"	136–151	139–153
5'10"	140–155	143–158
5'11"	—	147–163
6'0"	—	151–168
6'1"	—	155–173
6'2"	—	160–178
6'3"	—	165–183

CIRCA 1990

This table was issued by the United States Departments of Agriculture and Health and Human Services in 1990. Men and women were grouped together and broken down by age, suggesting that it is desirable for women over 35 to gain weight.

HEIGHT	19 TO 34	35 & OVER
5'0"	97–128	108–138
5'1"	101–132	111–143
5'2"	104–137	115–148
5'3"	107–141	119–152
5'4"	111–146	122–157
5'5"	114–150	126–162
5'6"	118–155	130–167
5'7"	121–160	134–172
5'8"	125–164	138–178
5'9"	129–169	142–183
5'10"	132–174	146–188
5'11"	136–179	151–194
6'0"	140–184	155–199
6'1"	144–189	159–205
6'2"	148–195	164–210
6'3"	152–200	168–216
6'4"	156–205	172–222
6'5"	160–211	177–228
6'6"	164–216	182–234

Are You Obese, Overweight, or Just Plain Fat?

Are you in major denial? You can still fit into that size twelve. Size four-teen doesn't look too disgusting. Hey, maybe you are even a size ten. And of course you are the thinnest one at your weight-loss club. You don't even come close to looking like some of your old high school friends. You joined a gym and even went once or twice. You've got that treadmill with last year's *Cosmo* sitting on it. You are AWARE. Terrific. You get the awareness medal. Now let's see if you are one of the 98 million chubbies in the United States. Let's see how fat you really are.

Your Body Mass Index

This is a new way to determine whether you are in serious trouble and whether fat is shortening your life. The body mass index (BMI) is believed by many researchers to be one of the most accurate ways to deter-mine your healthy weight. Find your height in inches on the left scale. Now find your weight in pounds on the right scale. Draw a line between them. Where that line meets in the middle is your approximate BMI.

Men	**Women**
25+ overweight	25+ overweight
21 to 25 acceptable weight	19 to 25 acceptable weight
Below 21 underweight	Below 19 underweight

BODY MASS INDEX CHART

Determining your healthy weight by calculating your body mass index (a number based on height and weight) is not a task for the mathematically challenged. The table below simplifies the calculation. Draw a line from your height, on the left side of the table, to your weight, on the right side. The point at which that line crosses the center is your approximate body mass index.

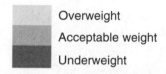

Overweight

Acceptable weight

Underweight

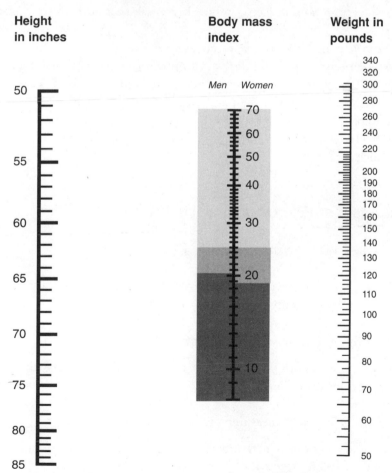

Height in inches   **Body mass index**   **Weight in pounds**

Source: *Journal of the American Dietetic Association*, September 1985.

> The Nurse's Health Study found that being of average weight, that is
> having a body mass index between 25 and 26.9, increases
> a woman's risk of dying prematurely by 30 percent.

Are You an Apple or a Pear?

Otherwise known as the waist-to-hip ratio (WHR) is another fat test that is enjoying a great deal of popularity for its accuracy in determining your fat zone and your risk of developing the diseases of premature aging. Scientists now believe that the location of fat deposits around your body is also a very important factor in how big a risk that fat is to your overall health.

Women generally have more fat around the hip area, making them pears. Men tend to have fat deposits around their middles, making them apples. The apples are at a greater risk for cardiovascular disease than the pears. So if you are a man and your WHR is greater than 1.0, you are an apple and too fat for your own health. If you are a woman and your WHR is more than 0.85, you're an apple too and are carrying way too much fat.

The Apple or Pear Do-It-Yourself Test

Here's the do-it-yourself version.

Using a fabric tape, measure your waist at the level of your belly button. Sucking in your tummy is cheating. Just stay relaxed.

1. My belly button waist measurement is_____

Now measure around your buttocks or hips. Find the place that's the widest and measure that.

2. My hip or buttocks measurement is _____

Now divide your hip measurement into your waist measurement or divide your second result into your first result.

My waist-to-hip ratio is _____

Now find your result on the chart and see where you fall in the risk category.

APPLE VS. PEAR RISK CHART

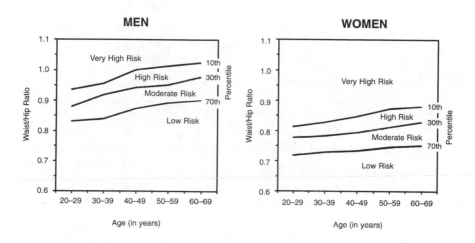

So Are You a Candidate for Losing Weight?

1. My BMI is greater than 30.
                    YES   NO
2. My waist-to-hip ratio is not good.
                    YES   NO
3. I have gained more than 15 pounds (women) or 10 pounds (men) since
   I was a teen or young adult.
                    YES   NO

Scoring: Even 1 YES makes you older and fatter before your time. Get on
the program, the *Fountain of Youth* program.

WHY WE GOT SO FAT IN THE FIRST PLACE

You guessed it. There are plenty of exotic theories around. Here are some of the new and trendy ones:

The Fat Antenna Proteins and the Obesity (ob) Gene

Certain proteins called leptin receptors give off a fullness signal that tells us when to stop eating. The ability to read these signals is housed in a "fat" gene. For many of us these signals get scrambled when faced with a chocolate chip cookie.

GLP-1

This is a powerful appetite suppressant that gets rats to eat 95 percent less food and still feel full. Scientists believe that this element may exist in the hypothalamus, which regulates appetite and other basic behavior in humans. When it is out of whack, we overeat.

Menopause and Hormones

These are believed by some researchers to account for the extra fat post-menopausal women carry. Some studies show that women who received hormone replacement therapy developed less fat around their abdomens than women who didn't take any hormones.

Back to the Basics

But we can't really blame our increasing fat on genes, hormones, molecular theories, and shrinking glands.

The reality is we eat too much, we eat the wrong things, we don't exercise, and many of us just don't care anymore. We are trying to try, but we are getting increasingly frustrated and confused by too many conflicting nutritional messages. We are stressed out by work and family responsibilities. We barely have enough time to do the weekly shopping, much less try to figure out the assorted labels, pyramids, fat grams, and calories.

It's just too much. And the more we fret, the more we eat. And the more we eat, the greater our frustration becomes.

A recent survey of Americans by the Calorie Council found:

65 percent believe they are overweight.
24 percent say they are on a diet.
78 percent use low-calorie products at least once every couple of weeks.
88 percent use low-fat products regularly.
78 percent believe they are eating healthier than they were three years ago.

So what do we do? We join weight-loss clubs and clinics. We buy thousands of dollars of "diet" food. We order every kind of fat-burning piece of equipment offered on late night shopping TV.

Never mind the fact that with some part of our brain we know we are too fat and that it isn't good for us. Never mind that we would like to lose weight and reduce our risk of dying young. But how? How can we get our insides thinner, our blood pressure down, and our cholesterol under control when we can't even manage to get into that size ten?

Relax. It's going to be easy.

EATING OUR WAY TO BETTER HEALTH

Sounds like it can't work, doesn't it? But it can work and it does work. Here's how.

Obesity

Obesity is a killer all by itself without any added health risks. At the annual meeting of the American College of Sports Medicine researchers reported that even when they took high blood pressure, inactivity, and smoking into account, obese people still died younger.

Cancer

Diet is associated with up to 60 percent of cancers in women according to the Food and Nutrition Board of the National Academy of Sciences. And the National Research Council points to excess calories, especially those from fat, as the biggest cancer culprits.

Eating a diet rich in vegetables, the *Fountain of Youth* diet, can cut your breast cancer risk by as much as tenfold. If you lose the weight, you also reduce the risk.

Lung cancer risk is five times higher in women (and men) whose diets are high in saturated fat, this from a study by the National Cancer Institute.

Prostate cancer has been linked to a diet high in meat and potatoes and low in antioxidant vegetables.

Skin cancer research at Baylor College of Medicine in Houston found people who ate a typical American diet of 38 percent of calories from fat had ten times the recurrence rate of skin cancer as those who ate a *Fountain of Youth* low-fat (20 percent) diet.

---

10 extra pounds can increase your breast cancer risk by 23 percent.
15 extra pounds can increase your breast cancer risk by 37 percent.
20 extra pounds can increase your breast cancer risk by 52 percent.

Heart Disease

Almost 30 percent of all women and 50 percent of women over fifty-five are at risk for heart disease. Heart disease kills 500,000 women a year and almost 40 percent of women who have a heart attack will die within the first year. Changes in eating habits and nutrition can save your life. The American Heart Association blames fat for most of the coronary heart disease. Studies of antioxidants are also proving that nutrients can extend your life expectancy. And a new study from the University of Maryland says that weight loss may be the most effective way to improve coronary artery disease risk factors. Gaining weight isn't so good for your heart either. Women who gained between twenty-four and forty-one pounds as adults doubled their risk of heart disease.

Osteoporosis

The American Dietetic Association says that good nutrition, such as adequate calcium, can help prevent the onset of osteoporosis and reduce the severity of the disorder. Osteoporosis is blamed for 1.5 million fractures a year and affects 25 million Americans.

High Blood Pressure

Studies show that on the average, blood pressure increases 6.5 systolic points (the upper number representing arterial pressure between beats) for men and 3.25 systolic points for women with every ten pounds of weight gain. On the other side of that coin, weight loss can dramatically reduce high blood pressure. Scientists estimate that losing twenty to twenty-five pounds can reduce your blood pressure, both systolic and diastolic, an average of eight to ten points.

Arthritis

Over 23 million women suffer from arthritis. The Centers for Disease Control in Atlanta cite weight control as one of the ways to control this painful chronic condition. And researchers at Loma Linda University School of Medicine found that eating more vegetarian-type meals helped relieve much of the pain.

Alzheimer's

Countless new studies point to the fact that diet may play a significant part in the development of senility and other aging disorders of the brain.

Diabetes

The risk for developing adult onset diabetes is three times greater for overweight folks as it is for those whose weight is where it should be.

Vision

According to the American Foundation for the Blind, everyone over the age of sixty-five suffers some vision loss: cataracts, macular degeneration, night blindness. What's a fix? Researchers have found those who eat a diet rich in antioxidants, like the one in *Fountain of Youth,* had half the risk for developing at least one of these eye problems—macular degeneration. Another study found that a high-fat diet increased the risk of blindness by 80 percent.

Lung Disorders

Fountain of Youth antioxidants impact directly on lung function. A joint EPA-Harvard study found that lung function and vitamin C intake from fruits and vegetables were directly related.

Depression

In a large-scale study over 500 women cut their dietary fat by 50 percent for twelve months. The results? They experienced less anxiety, stress, and depression and reported feeling more energized and invigorated.

Sore Feet

Fat hurts your feet. A study from the University of California found that women who were 20 percent above their ideal weight had more inflammation and pain in their heels and arches, more tendinitis, ankle sprains, and broken bones.

ESCHEW OBFUSCATION

I once saw a terrific T-shirt that said ESCHEW OBFUSCATION. I had to look it up—both words. It means "eliminate confusion." And that's what happens next. Forget everything you were ever told about calories, fat grams, pyramid power, labels, portions, and RDAs. You don't have time. And much of that nutritional mumbo jumbo is so confusing it's hurting you more than helping you. For those of you with a scientific bent, all that "stuff" is listed at the back of this book in the glossary.

First of all, *Fountain of Youth* is like no other weight-loss program you have ever been on . . . or off . . . or on and off. Everything is done for you. All you have to do is turn each page and eat.

Going grocery shopping? Great. With the *Fountain of Youth* all you have to do is turn the page and buy.

Your turn to cook? No sweat. It's either broil, bake, grill, or steam. How hard can that be?

Out of something? No problem. If you've got something green, orange, red, or yellow in your fridge, you can add it, substitute it, or even double it. Just don't forget it.

After you get through the core program you will be so good at picking just the right stuff, you won't need charts, graphs, scales, calculators, tables, slide rules, or Dick Tracy watches to shop, cook, or eat properly.

GETTING OUT THE FAT, PUTTING IN THE THIN

Fountain of Youth is not about dieting at all. It isn't about what you can't eat, shouldn't eat, musn't eat. Forget the guilt. This is about what you should eat, must eat, have to eat, want to eat, to get younger, healthier, and thinner. This is the only program that tells you—EAT!

STOP STARVING TO DEATH

Whether you are on a flavor-of-the-month diet or still chowing down on burgers and fries, you are starving to death. Every one of your 50 trillion cells is swimming in a sticky fat soup and is starving for nutrition. And let's face it, another hamburger, another soda, even another nonfat dessert isn't going to feed those cells. Give them a break. Give those poor little molecules some vitamin C, a shot of vitamin E, a generous helping of beta-carotene, some calcium. Stop committing nutritional suicide. Stop killing yourself cell by cell, and start pumping some life force into your body.

What will happen when you do? When you fill yourself with nutrient-dense foods, foods chock-full of fountain of youth vitamins and minerals, there won't be any room for fat. And when there's no room for fat, what happens? Your body gets thinner. So you are going to do something wonderful for yourself. You are going to eat your way to a younger, thinner, healthier you.

So, what are you waiting for? Let's go!

CHAPTER 3

How Old Are You Really?

How old would you be if you didn't know how old you was?
—SATCHEL PAIGE

That's a very good question. How old *would* you be if you really didn't know how old you were? Stop and think about that for a minute. What if your birth certificate had been destroyed in a fire? If your parents developed amnesia the day you were born? If you were suddenly dropped from a spaceship and found yourself wandering around the mall?

THE CALENDAR METHOD

Determining chronological age is a precise science. Formulas tabulate the number of hours in a day, the number of days in a week, weeks in a month, months in a year. Then the calendar cycle starts all over again. And as the count changes another year is recorded against our age. This is the tried-and-true calendar method of determining the passage of time and with it determining age. It is a very useful method if you are setting tax deadlines, applying for social security benefits, stringing decorations for national holidays, buying gifts for anniversaries, marking the start of the hunting season, or deciding when to plant your tomatoes. But is the chronological or calendar method reliable in fixing our true age? Are there other, perhaps more accurate ways, to determine how old we are? Stick around, you will be surprised.

THE MIRROR METHOD

This is a good one. It's not very scientific, but it has the benefit of shock value. Here's how it works.

Have you ever suddenly surprisingly found yourself in front of a mirror (or a plate-glass window), glanced at the image, and saw—your mother? (or your father?) Saw that you looked older than you thought you were? Wasn't that a shock? Didn't a little of the spring go out of your step? Didn't you make a mental note to get that checkup you've been putting off? Didn't you think for just a moment about liposuction or even a face-lift?

Or have you ever come upon a mirror you weren't expecting and saw the reflection of a youthful, smiling face, and a slender figure, then, only a second or two later, realized it was your own. You looked thin and stylish. Wasn't that a pleasant surprise? Didn't you decide to treat yourself to that new lipstick you thought was maybe too bright for an "old lady" like you? Didn't you think that maybe tonight that sexy nightie you put away should come out of its box? Or that maybe it really wasn't too late to take up tennis?

The power of the mirror and what we see in it is one way we determine how old we would be if we didn't know how old we were.

THE MILESTONE METHOD

Here's another one. This is one that brings us up short from time to time. Picture this scenario. You worked all day. Then you stopped off at the supermarket. You drove home through rush hour traffic, threw some dinner on for the two kids, did a load of laundry. So far a pretty typical day. Now here's the difference. Here comes the age marker. Ready? Instead of curling up with the ironing or a bowl of popcorn and a movie from the local video store you find the energy to shower, change, dig out your sparkling earrings, and go out with your main squeeze to celebrate your twenty-fifth wedding anniversary. There you both are. A bottle of champagne cools in a bucket beside you. A fragrant bowl of pasta steams garlic. A candle drips wax down a bottle of Chianti. You are back in the little Italian (it's always Italian) restaurant where you met. You look at him. He looks at you and you can't believe that the boy you married is fifty. You do the same fast math. If he's fifty that makes you forty-seven. And in the years between your first date and this one you have produced three kids, one of whom is almost twenty-five years old and about to make you a grandmother. You know you don't look old enough to be celebrating twenty-five years together and you certainly don't feel old enough either. And yet there is the milestone, a major anniversary.

The milestone method jumps up and hits us hard between the years, most particularly on special occasions of so-called milestone birthdays when we slam against the rock of age and leave the encounter shaken. If there were no milestones, how old would we think we were?

THE BIRTHDAY CANDLE METHOD

How many birthday candles did you blow out on your last birthday cake? Thirty? Thirty-five? Forty? Fifty? Or did you do what I started to do a dozen birthdays ago and just put one great big candle smack in the middle of the cake and start eating around it?

This tradition of blowing out more and more candles with less and less lung power is one of the more ridiculous and humiliating ways to count off the passing years. It is particularly odious when coupled with people wearing funny hats and leaping up yelling, "Surprise!"

If there was no birthday cake, if there were no candles, how old would you be?

THE DENIAL METHOD

This is a great system for measuring your true age and my personal favorite. You simply pick the age you want and stay there.

THE YEARBOOK METHOD

This one is really fun. You get a letter, usually the day you move up one dress size, with an invitation to your high school reunion. We all know what happens then. Out come the yearbooks. After a pleasant two hours or so of tripping down memory lane you realize with a panic that you can't possibly go. You don't have time to lose those thirty pounds that snuck up on you since graduation. There aren't enough cucumbers or tea bags in the country to smooth your puffy eyelids or make the dark circles and bags under your eyes vanish. The laugh lines that looked so cute in that prom photo have settled into wrinkles and your bosom is no longer where it used to be. Oh, sure, your neighbors think you look great. The boy at the checkout counter gives you an appreciative glance when he loads your groceries. And you just got that promotion. But deep down inside you know you won't pass the scrutiny of your high school friends. You see yourself through their eyes and suddenly you are older.

If there was no reunion, if there was no yearbook, how old would you be, do you think?

THE BIOLOGICAL METHOD OR ARE YOU "WEARING OUT" TOO SOON?

Now we come to the true method of determining just how old we really are. While the calendar measures the actual number of years we have lived and the mirror reflects how we look, and the milestones, candles, and yearbooks give us clues as to how we have changed, longevity scientists have devised another more exciting and more exact way to measure our true age. Is our body older or younger than the calendar? Is it older or younger than the mirror shows? Is it older or younger than all the milestones, candles, and yearbooks measure? You'll soon see for yourself.

THE THREE AGES OF MAN

CHRONOLOGICAL AGE—how old you are by the calendar.
BIOLOGICAL AGE—how old your body is in terms of critical life signs and cellular processes.
PSYCHOLOGICAL AGE—how old you feel you are.

—Ageless Body, Timeless Mind by DEEPAK CHOPRA

IT ALL STARTED WHEN BOOMERS WORE DIAPERS

In the 1950s, when the first baby boomers were graduating to training pants and leaving strained baby food behind forever, researchers began to look for the secret to measuring biological age. They wondered why some people were doing the limbo on cruise ships at sixty while others were gray, dismal, set in their ways, and old at forty. Why, they asked, were some thirty-year-olds, as measured by the calendar, old before their years and some winning marathons? Why, they asked, were some fifty-year-olds enjoying vigorous second, third, and even fourth honeymoons, while others of the same calendar age are shuffling around in ratty robes, unable to remember the last time they enjoyed the crunch of an apple, the thrill of an adventure, or the warm satisfaction of making love?

And so they began to look for the clues beyond the seasons, the anniversaries and the calendar that would unlock the secrets of true age. What were these magic measurements? Was there a pattern? And most importantly, could these measurements of true age be manipulated? Could the relentless clock of nature be forced to run backwards, away from the linear measure of time and back into the biological state of youth?

It was in Canada that a major breakthrough was finally made. Around the time that the Beatles were shattering our views of music and flower power was mightier than guns, Dr. Robert Morgan devised a standardized test for measuring biological age. He called this instrument the Adult Growth Examination (AGE) and his is the distinction of formulating one of the most accurate ways for us to determine how old we really are. Dr. Morgan's test involved only three simple measurements based on physiology: blood pressure, near-vision blurring, and high-frequency hearing.

In the ensuing years other scientists added to this test and discovered other body function measurements of age. In the mid-1980s researchers at the Canadian Institute of Stress modified these measurements and in a remarkable study tested 623 people who measured biologically older than their calendar age by as much as ten years or more. They then went on to show that these subjects could reverse their personal march of time, cheat the calendar, fool the clock, and become younger—not just younger by a year or two, but younger by ten, twenty, and even twenty-five years! Their findings are mind-boggling:

- You *can* reduce your biological age, or body age.
- You *can* look younger.
- You *can* feel better.
- Although premature or accelerated aging can take place at any stage of life, it is most prevalent among people in their prime.
- People in their fifties and sixties are as able to lower their body ages as people in their thirties or forties.

Over the next decade others would add to this research so that today we are able, without expensive equipment, complicated formulas, and complex testing methods, to determine for ourselves, in the privacy of our own homes, exactly how old we are.

WHY BOTHER FINDING YOUR TRUE BIOLOGICAL AGE?

Curiosity. Fear. Hope. Without the facts, without knowing how old you really are, you can't adjust your own biological clock. How can you set your alarm clock to wake you up at a certain time if you don't now what time it is when you activate the ringer? How can you know how long your cookies have to bake if you don't know what time you first put them in the oven? How do you know when to start supper if you don't know when your guests will arrive? How much more important to know exactly where you are starting from, where the hands of your very own biological clock are right now, this minute, in order to turn them back to fifty, forty, thirty, even twenty?

Our body is a well-set clock, which keeps good time, but if it be too much or indiscreetly tampered with, the alarm runs out before the hour.

—JOSEPH HALL

And believe me, most of us want to be younger. I know I wanted it. We want the energy, the vigor, the glow that we had two, ten, or even twenty years ago. We want the agility, the health, the posture, the flame that burns so brightly in a youthful body and flickers and dims in an aging one. I know I did. We want to finally win the battle of the bulging waistline that seems almost an inevitability of age. I know I did.

That's how I started. With research and more research until I found the very best, simplest, and most understandable aging tests available. I did them. I measured my own age. And as a result I was able to count in double digits (that's in the tens plus) the number of years that dropped away and the pounds that disappeared. These tests were my beginning. They must be yours. Without these tests you will not be able to fully experience the program. You won't be able to appreciate the progress you have made. You won't have an accurate record of just how much younger and thinner you have become. You won't enjoy the new you that will emerge years younger and pounds thinner and healthier from the *Fountain of Youth*.

ABOUT THE FOUNTAIN OF YOUTH TESTS

The tests included in this chapter have proven to be accurate, simple, and true in thousands of research hours, dozens of laboratories, and hundreds of studies. I have examined the research data for you and pulled those tests that can be done quickly at home without any special equipment and at little cost to you.

No one compiles data such as this alone, and I'm no exception. I had a lot of help from some very knowledgeable folks. Two wonderful Canadian researchers wrote a book called *Your Vitality Quotient* (Warner Books, 1989). They were really the ones who got my own juices flowing about my personal potential for youth and who first introduced me to the shock of determining my own true biological age. Once these two innovative scientists got me started, there was no holding me back. Other tests were adapted from such books as *Controlling Cholesterol* (Bantam Books, 1988) by Kenneth Cooper, M.D., and *Biomarkers* (Simon & Schuster, 1991) by William Evans, M.D., and Irwin Hosenberg, M.D., as well as many, many others. Go for it. Become your own biological detective. I guarantee you won't be disappointed and the journey will be the most interesting one you will ever take.

But enough about tests in general. Let's talk for a moment about the weight test in particular. This test is the one that I most dreaded and I know you probably do too. But remember, it is very important, because weight is very closely tied into premature aging. The weight test affects so much of your physiology and extra pounds seriously increase your risk for life-shortening diseases such as heart disease, stroke, osteoporosis, and diabetes. The extra age you carry with extra pounds puts a strain on your joints and your organs and reduces your ability to enjoy a youthful quality of life.

So when you take these *Fountain of Youth* tests remember, they are the pass to the *Fountain of Youth: The Anti-Aging Weight-Loss Program.* They are your tickets to a whole new, healthy life.

THE TESTS YOU WILL BE DOING

Test #1 The Skin Pinch Bio-Test
Test #2 The Resting Heart Rate Bio-Test
Test #3 The Big Blur or Visual Acuity Bio-Test
Test #4 The Systolic Blood Pressure Bio-Test
Test #5 The Cholesterol Bio-Test
Test #6 The Weight Bio-Test

GETTING STARTED

Don't be scared. Think of this as a wonderful adventure. Once you do these few simple tests you will have completed the very first step in getting younger every day. You will have a true measurement of how old you really are. You will be able to set youth-enhancement goals that you will reach. You will stop thinking of birthdays as markers of age and will start thinking of them as indicators of youth. You will no longer be a slave to the calendar, the mirror, the milestone, the birthday cake, the yearbook. You will have broken the barriers of age as it has been known and measured for centuries past and will have entered the exciting new world of longevity.

GETTING THE "STUFF" YOU NEED TOGETHER

Before you begin you will need a few very simple items, many of which you probably already have around the house.

A Blood Pressure Monitor

You can get one of these at any pharmacy and they come in a variety of types and at a variety of price ranges. You need this for one of the most important tests of biological age and you will need it ninety days later when you test yourself younger after you have completed this program. If you don't want to go to the expense of purchasing your own blood pressure monitor, get your blood pressure checked by your doctor or health professional. Many places offer free blood pressure screenings and will help you write down your blood pressure accurately.

A Watch with a Sweep Second Hand

A digital watch or clock won't work for these tests. We are going to be taking measurements in exact seconds so find yourself one of the old-fashioned watches that lets you monitor each and every second.

A Yardstick

If you do a lot of sewing you probably have one of these near your sewing machine. It is important that you get the wooden kind that you can pick up in any hardware store. Don't use the kind that is made of cloth and rolls up in a ball.

A Metal Tape Measure

We all have one of these somewhere. Mine is usually in my kitchen junk drawer. But if you are more organized, yours is probably in the toolbox where it belongs. If you don't have one you can easily get a small one in any hardware store and even in the hardware department of most grocery stores.

A 3 x 5-Inch File Card

You know the type I mean. These are the cards that are usually lined on one side and plain on the other. Most of us use them to write down our favorite recipes and store them in a file box. Find a blank one or buy a small packet in any stationery store. You could also try your grocery store in the same section as writing paper, Scotch tape, and crayons.

A Cholesterol Testing Home Kit

Purchase a cholesterol testing kit from your local pharmacy or, if you prefer, have your doctor or other health professional take your cholesterol level and give you the results.

An Accurate Bathroom Scale

I hate to tell you this, but one of the aging tests is directly tied to your weight so you will need an accurate bathroom scale. Sorry. But you will thank me later.

A Notepad and a Pen

You will need a sheet of paper to record all your scores. I suggest using a pen; that way you won't be tempted to rub out scores and cheat.

That's it. That's all the equipment you will need to determine your own biological or body age. Nothing too sophisticated. Nothing too complicated. Nothing too intimidating.

THE BUDDY SYSTEM

Find yourself a buddy and do the tests together. You can do some of these body age tests all by yourself. But there are a couple where you are going to need a little help. In fact, besides being a great help in recording body age scores, doing it with a buddy turns this exercise into a lot of fun. If you are embarrassed you don't have to share scores. You can keep your own private and hidden until the ninety days goes by and then you can see which of you got younger and by how much.

Who to pick for your buddy? Pick a friend. Pick your spouse. Get a group together and turn this into an anti-aging project. You and your buddy don't need any special skills or knowledge. All you need is the desire to become younger, slimmer, and healthier.

You can do these tests in any order.
Now, on your mark, get set,
go!

IMPORTANT: BEFORE YOU BEGIN

1. Check with your doctor before you undertake any of these tests.
2. Some of the tests offer a range of ages. I suggest that you either average the range or take the highest number in the range as your body age. For example, if the body age is expressed as a range from thirty to forty, either average those two figures together to get thirty-five and use that number as the body age resulting from the test, or take the highest number, in our example forty, as the body age resulting from the test.

TEST #I THE SKIN PINCH BIO-TEST

What You Will Need

- A table or desk top
- A comfortable chair
- A watch or clock with a sweep second hand

What This Test Measures

This test measures the elasticity of your skin. Why is this an indicator of body age? As we get older our skin, which is the largest organ in the body, loses its youthful resilience. This test is one of the best indicators of the biological age of this very visible organ and a foreshadowing of wrinkles. Wrinkles begin in the dermis, the layer of tissue below the visible surface of the skin. This layer is bursting with blood vessels, nerve endings, and glands that feed the surface layer, keeping it soft and supple. As our body ages, the dermis stiffens and shrinks. The stiffening of the connective tissues in the dermis and the shrinking cause the surface layer of skin to loosen and fall in an irregular pattern. The dips and grooves in the pattern are the wrinkles we see as we age.

Ready, Set, Go

Sit down in your chair and pull it up to the surface of a table or desk. Get your sweep second hand watch ready. Now, place one hand, palm down, on the surface of the table. It doesn't matter which hand you choose. Keep your hand relaxed. With the thumb and forefinger of the other hand pinch a large piece of skin from the middle of the flat, relaxed hand. Here's where the seconds come in. Hold the pinched skin firmly for a count of five seconds. Release. Count the number of seconds it takes for the pinched skin to go back to normal.

Figuring Out Your Score

> NOTE: In this test the scoring is the same for men and women.

Using the chart below, find the number of seconds it took your skin to go back to normal, flat. That's in the first column. Then find your corresponding body age in years. That's in the second column. Write down your score. If you like you can repeat the test on the other hand and then take the average as your final score.

Skin Elasticity in Seconds	Body Age in Years
0 to 2	19
2 to 4	30
4 to 6	40
6 to 8	45
8 to 10	50
10 to 12	60
12 to 14	70+

My Personal Score

Skin Elasticity in Seconds:_____

Body Age in Years: _____

My body age in the skin pinch test is: _____

TEST #2 THE RESTING HEART RATE BIO-TEST

What You Will Need

- A comfortable chair
- A watch or clock with a sweep second hand

What This Test Measures

This test measures the ability of your heart to pump oxygen-rich blood into your system, allowing you the health and vigor to exercise and lead an active life. In dozens of studies researchers found that our ability to transport oxygen declines as our body age increases. This decrease begins in our thirties (for men it starts earlier, in their twenties) and continues through our adult years until by age sixty-five we have 30 to 40 percent less invigorating oxygen in our muscles than we had as teenagers. The famous Framingham Study, which followed 2,400 women since 1949, found that women have a ten-year edge on their male counterparts in terms of heart disease. But, the shocking news was that even though women can buy themselves an extra ten years before the onset of aging heart disease, they don't benefit as much as men if they wait to take some preventive measures after they have been diagnosed with heart problems. This test can measure the age of your heart and can help you take steps to make it younger and healthier before it is too late.

Ready, Set, Go

Sit down in your comfortable chair. Put your watch with the sweep second hand in front of you where you can see it clearly. Don't hold your breath. Relax. Now find your pulse by putting your middle finger on the large artery in your throat, just under your chin. Put your fingers on that artery gently. Too much pressure can cut off some of the blood flow. If you have trouble finding the pulse under your chin you can use the pulse on the inside of your wrist. If you are going to use your wrist pulse, pull your chair up to a table or desk and place your arm comfortably on the surface. Then locate your pulse. Wait until you're sure you have it. Now start counting and watching the sweep second hand. Count the number of pulses in twenty seconds. Repeat the count a couple of times more so that you're sure it's accurate. Now multiply the number of pulses you counted by three. This gives you your resting heart rate for one minute.

> WARNING: Do not use your thumb to count out your pulses. Your thumb has a pulse of its own, which will skew your result.

Figuring Out Your Score

Using the chart below, find the number of beats per minute you timed in the first column. Then find your corresponding body age in years. That's in the second column. Write down your score.

FOR WOMEN ONLY

Heart Rate Beats per Minute	Body Age in Years
50 or less to 62	19
63	20
64	22
65	25
66	27
67	30
68	33
69	35
70	37
71	39
72	41
73	43
74	45
75	46
76	47
77	48
78	49
79	50
80	51
81	52
82	53
83	54
84	55
85	58
86	60
87 to 88	63
89 to 90	64
91 to 92	65
93 to 95	66
96 to 97	67
98	68
99	69
100 plus	71 plus

FOR MEN ONLY

Heart Rate Beats per Minute	Body Age in Years
50 or less to 60	19
61	20
62	21
63	24
64	27
65	30
66	32
67	35
68	38
69	40
70	42
71	44
72	46
73	48
74	50
75	51
76	52
77	53
78	54
79	55
80	56
81	57
82	58
83	59
84	60
85	63
86	65
87	67
88	69
89	71
90	72
91	73
92	74
93	76
94	77
95	78 plus

My Personal Score

Heart Rate in Beats Per Minute:_____

Body Age in Years:_____

My body age in the resting heart rate test is:_____

TEST #3 THE BIG BLUR OR VISUAL ACUITY BIO-TEST

What You Will Need

- A 3 x 5-inch index card
- A metal tape measure
- A buddy

What This Test Measures

As we age, the lens in our eye begins to become less pliable and loses its elasticity. This test is one indicator of how much elasticity we may have already lost.

Ready, Set, Go

> I Will Get Younger Every Day

Type the sentence in the box in the middle of your index card. Use a standard typewriter with 10-pica type. This is a pretty standard type for most typewriters so you shouldn't have any trouble. Tape the card to the end of the scrolling metal tape measure so that it stands up and the typed side is facing you. Now place the tape casing against your cheek under your

right eye. Make sure that the typed side is facing you. This is very important. Cover your left eye with your other hand. Now get your buddy to
pull the end of the tape measure with the attached card out in front of you
until it is six feet away. Then have your buddy walk toward you, slowly
scrolling the tape back into its casing. You watch the card closely. When
the letters begin to blur make a note of the distance between you and the
card. Do the same test with your other eye. Then take the average of the
two numbers.

NOTE: Don't wear your glasses or contact lenses for this test.

Figuring Out Your Score

NOTE: In this test the scoring is the same for men and women.

Using the chart below, find the number of inches in the first column that
correspond to the place at which your vision blurred. Remember to use
the average of both eyes. Then, in the second column, find the corresponding biological or body age.

Near Vision in Inches	Body Age in Years
0 to 3.9	19
4.0 to 4.1	20
4.2	21
4.3	22
4.4 to 4.5	23
4.6 to 4.7	24
4.8	25
4.9 to 5.0	26
5.1	27
5.2 to 5.3	28
5.4	29
5.5 to 5.7	30

Near Vision in Inches			Body Age in Years
5.8	to	6.1	31
6.2	to	6.5	32
6.6	to	6.8	33
6.9	to	7.1	34
7.2	to	7.5	35
7.6	to	7.9	36
8.0	to	8.2	37
8.3	to	8.5	38
8.6	to	8.9	39
9.0	to	9.5	40
9.6	to	10.1	41
10.2	to	10.7	42
10.8	to	11.3	43
11.4	to	11.9	44
12	to	12.5	45
12.6	to	13.1	46
13.2	to	13.7	47
13.8	to	14.3	48
14.4	to	14.9	49
15	to	17.3	50
17.4	to	19.7	51
19.8	to	22.1	52
22.2	to	24.5	53
24.6	to	26.9	54
27	to	29.3	55
29.4	to	31.7	56
31.8	to	34.1	57
34.2	to	36.5	58
36.6	to	38.9	59
39	to	41.3	60
41.4	to	43.7	61
43.8	to	46.1	62
46.2	to	48.5	63
48.6	to	50.9	64
51	to	53.3	65
53.4	to	55.7	66
55.8	to	58.1	67
58.2	to	60.5	68
60.6	to	62.9	69
63	to	65.3	70

My Personal Score

Near Vision in Inches: _____

Body Age in Years: _____

My body age in the big blur test is: _____

Don't despair about your big blur test results. Even if you are as blind as the proverbial bat, this isn't the be-all and end-all and this result will not lock you into a biological age that can't be altered.

TEST #4 THE SYSTOLIC BLOOD PRESSURE BIO-TEST

What You Will Need

- A recent blood pressure reading or a home blood pressure monitor

What This Test Measures

Blood pressure is one of the major indicators of our biological age. Blood pressure is always shown in two numbers, one on top of the other. The top number measures the pressure in your blood vessels when your heart is pumping and is called the systolic pressure. The lower number measures the pressure when your heart is at rest and is called the diastolic. Both numbers are important indicators of your heart and blood vessel health. But the systolic number is the one used in age tests.

Ready, Set, Go

If you have your recent blood pressure from your doctor or from another health professional, use only the top or first number, the systolic measurement. If you have a home blood pressure monitor take your blood pressure following the directions exactly. Make a note of your blood pressure and again use only the top number.

Figuring Out Your Score

Using the chart below, find the number that corresponds to the first number or upper number of your blood pressure in the first column. Then find the body age that matches.

NOTE: Men and women have different readings. If you are a woman taking this test, use the chart for women. If you are a man taking this test, use the chart for men.

FOR WOMEN ONLY

Systolic Blood Pressure	Body Age in Years
0 to 110	19 or less
111	20
112	21
113	23
114	25
115	28
116	30
117	32
118	33
119	35
120	36
121	37
122	39
123	40

Systolic Blood Pressure	Body Age in Years
124	41
125	42
126	43
127	44
128	45
129 to 130	46
131	47
132	48
133	49
134	50
135	52
136	53
137	55
138	56
139	58
140 to 141	59
142 to 143	61
144 to 145	62
146 to 147	63
148 to 149	64
150 to 151	65
152 to 153	66
154 to 155	67
156 to 157	68
158 to 159	69
160	70

FOR MEN ONLY

Systolic Blood Pressure	Body Age in Years
0 to 120	19 or less
121	20
122	21
123	24
124	27
125	30
126	32
127	35

Systolic Blood Pressure	Body Age in Years
128	38
129	40
130	42
131	44
132	46
133	48
134	50
135	51
136	52
137	53
138	54
139	55
140	56
141	57
142	58
143	59
144	60
145	63
146	65
147	67
148	69
149	71

My Personal Score

Systolic Blood Pressure: _____

Body Age in Years: _____

My body age in the systolic blood pressure test is: _____

People whose systolic blood pressure is slightly above normal face increased health risk. The Physicians' Health Study at Brigham and Women's Hospital in Boston found that those whose systolic pressure was 140 to 159 had a 61 percent higher risk of death from heart disease and a 68 percent higher risk of stroke, compared to people whose systolic pressure was normal (under 140).

TEST #5 THE CHOLESTEROL BIO-TEST

What You Will Need

• A recent cholesterol reading from your physician or health professional or a home cholesterol testing kit.

What This Test Measures

Cholesterol is a fatty substance that sticks to the insides of our blood vessels, making them narrower. This means that our hearts have to pump harder in order to get youth-enhancing nutrients to the rest of our body. While HDL (good cholesterol), LDL (bad cholesterol), and the ratio between them are very important factors, this test concentrates on total cholesterol as an indicator of the bio-age of our arteries.

Ready, Set, Go

If you have your cholesterol readings from your physician or health professional, use the total cholesterol level for this test. If you have completed a home test for cholesterol, follow the instructions exactly and use only the total cholesterol number.

Figuring Out Your Score

Using the charts below, find the number that is closest to your cholesterol level in the first column. Now go across to the corresponding age range. Write down your score.

FOR WOMEN ONLY

Total Cholesterol Level	Age
179	Under 30
186	30 to 39
194	40 to 49
219	50 to 59
221	60 plus

FOR MEN ONLY

Total Cholesterol Level	Age
179	Under 30
191	30 to 39
205	40 to 49
208	50 to 59
208	60 plus

My Personal Score

Total cholesterol: _____

Age range: _____

My body age in the cholesterol test is: _____

> The ratio between "good" and "bad" cholesterol is very important. But for now this one will do as an age indicator.

TEST #6 THE WEIGHT BIO-TEST

What You Will Need

- An accurate scale
- A tape measure to measure your height

What This Test Measures

This one is easy. It measures your weight and height and correlates them to an age scale. Overweight and obesity are important factors in premature aging, so don't skip this one. If you like, you may take your weight at different times of the day and then average them out to get one number.

Ready, Set, Go

Stand up straight without your shoes on and wearing light clothing. Now have your buddy measure your height with the metal tape measure. Jot down your height. Next, step on your scale. Jot down your weight. That's all there is. Simple.

Figuring Out Your Score

Using the chart, find your height in the first column. Then find your ideal weight for your height.

Two Special Things You Should Know About This Test

1. Don't be shocked by what your weight says your age should be. When I took this test, the weights for both men and women skewed higher. Medical authorities believed that it was normal and healthy to gain weight with age. In the mid-1990s changes were made yet again to the healthy weight ranges for men and women as set out in the dietary guidelines for Americans. These are set at a much lower rate. Still, not all experts agree with the new ranges. And so the controversy rages on.
2. Some of you might think that if you are, say, 5'6" and weigh 141 pounds that makes you a blimp. However, before you pat yourself on the back for weighing in less than the minimums on this test remember over 50 percent of Americans are not just overweight, but obese. There are many of us out there who are 5'6" tall and weigh well over 150, 160, and even over 200 pounds. And fatter is

older. Also, this is but one test among many. Even if your body is thin, how are your arteries, your muscles, your joints?

How to Read Your Score

Find your height in the left-hand column. Move your finger along the line from your height to the right and find the column in which your weight in pounds falls. Now move your finger up the column to the top to find out just how old (or young) your weight makes you.

FOR WOMEN ONLY

Height	Age Ranges				
	18–24	25–34	35–44	45–54	55–64
4' 10"	114	123	133	132	135+
4' 11"	118	126	136	136	138+
5' 0"	121	130	139	139	142+
5' 1"	124	133	141	143	145+
5' 2"	128	136	144	146	148+
5' 3"	131	139	146	150	151+
5' 4"	134	142	149	153	154+
5' 5"	137	146	151	157	157+
5' 6"	141	149	154	160	161+
5' 7"	144	154	156	164	164+
5' 8"	147	155	159	168	167+

FOR MEN ONLY

Height	Age Ranges				
	18–24	25–34	35–44	45–54	55–64
5' 2"	130	139	146	148	147+
5' 3"	135	145	149	154	151+
5' 4"	139	151	155	158	156+
5' 5"	143	155	159	163	160+
5' 6"	148	159	164	167	165+
5' 7"	152	164	169	171	170+

Height	Age Ranges				
	18–24	25–34	35–44	45–54	55–64
5' 8"	157	168	174	176	174+
5' 9"	162	173	178	180	178+
5' 10"	166	177	183	185	183+
5' 11"	171	182	188	190	187+
6'	175	186	192	194	192+
6' 1"	180	191	197	198	197+
6' 2"	185	196	202	204	201+

My body age in the weight test is: _____

ABOUT EDITA'S SCORE

When I first did this test I weighed 168 pounds and I was 5'6" tall.
This put my biological age in the fifty-five to sixty-four year range.
Ninety days later I weighed 148 pounds.
Since I didn't shrink or grow taller, my biological age was reduced to
the 25- to 34-year range!

Developing Your own Bio-Age Profile

Here comes the fun part. Here is where you find out exactly how old your
body really is. This is your next step to a younger, thinner you. No matter
what your score don't be discouraged. If you come out one, two, five, ten,
or even more years older, we will change all this together. If you come out
at the exact same age as the calendar says you are you can get years
younger and pounds thinner. And even if you come out a few years
younger than your birthdays indicate you can still push back the clock
and become even slimmer and more youthful than you are now. So let's
do some simple math and add up the scores, divide them by the number
of tests, and see how old you really are. Ready?

Beside each test write down your personal body age.

Test #1 The Skin Pinch Bio-Test Score_____

Test #2 The Resting Heart Rate Bio-Test Score_____

Test #3 The Big Blur or Visual Acuity Bio-Test Score_____

Test #4 The Systolic Blood Pressure Bio-Test Score_____

Test #5 The Cholesterol Bio-Test Score_____

Test #6 The Weight Bio-Test Score_____

Now add up the totals of all the scores:_____

Divide this number by 6. This final number is your bio-age right now.

My bio-age is: _____

What's Next?

Now that you've completed the *Fountain of Youth* tests and have an accurate picture of where you are in terms of your age, you are ready to begin. Then, in a short and exciting ninety days, you will come back to this chapter and redo your tests. And guess what? You too will be younger, thinner, and healthier by far.

PART TWO

ANTIOXIDANTS:
THE YOUTH NUTRIENTS

CHAPTER 4

Youth Nutrients

As I see it, every day you do one of two things: Build health or produce disease in yourself.

—ADELLE DAVIS

A RADICAL REVIEW

For the want of a nail the shoe was lost,
For the want of a shoe the horse was lost,
For the want of a horse the rider was lost,
For the want of a rider the battle was lost,
For the want of a battle the kingdom was lost,
And all for the want of a horse-shoe nail.

Benjamin Franklin, remember him, he's the one with the kite, wrote these lines a very long time ago. He was writing about the irony of small, seemingly insignificant things, things we don't even notice, bringing down the mightiest creations of God and man. He probably sat there with a quill pen and scrap of parchment looking out the window at the early stirrings of that very storm.

But Ben might as well have been writing these lines yesterday on a computer while watching a split screen TV because the same principle is at work. Small, invisible, seemingly insignificant things can and do cause the destruction of the greatest of all the great natural wonders—us. You and me, and the local news anchor, and that funny waiter, and the drive-through bank teller, and the celebrity on your favorite talk show, and the list goes on and on.

So what is this small, seemingly insignificant thing that is working its destruction even as I write this and even as you read it? A free radical, that's what.

Remember those? Sure you do. But in case you've forgotten, here's a quick review. Free radicals are the by-products of normal metabolism—a kind of molecular garbage. Free radicals are produced when our bodies convert food into energy, when we fight off infections, when we are exposed to environmental pollutants such as cigarette smoke, exhaust fumes, and other toxic substances. Free radicals are produced when we take a walk, eat, go to the beach, eat, listen to music, eat, fix a tailgate spread, eat, make love, eat, nap, and eat. Free radicals are produced when we simply live and eat.

Free radicals are renegade substances. They are the great white sharks of the subatomic. These are not nice guys. Free radicals are molecules that are missing an electron, which makes them unstable. This makes them crazy. So what do they do? They rush around trying to steal an electron from some other molecule and in the process they bash into our fragile cell walls and tear apart normal atoms; they even damage the delicate genetic blueprint stored in our DNA. That's a lot of destruction. And we are getting hit with about ten thousand of these every single day.

Not everything these free radicals do is so very terrible. Some of it is actually pretty good. Without free radicals we wouldn't have plastic, bread wouldn't turn into toast, we wouldn't have any hydrogen peroxide (and so would have only natural blonds), we wouldn't have medicines that fight fungus like athlete's foot or that kill bacteria.

But the dark side of free radicals is what causes masterpieces to deteriorate, rubber to get brittle, cars to rust, apples to turn brown, butter to turn rancid, and us to age, sicken, and die.

THE OXYGEN PARADOX

Enter oxygen. We've all heard of this, right? So what does oxygen have to do with free radicals and premature aging and even getting fatter and getting thinner? I'm glad you asked that question. Because oxygen has an evil twin.

Picture the scene: an earth before time, a fiery ball hung in an inky sky. Almost 4 billion years ago when the earth was just a pot of space soup kept bubbling hot by the sun the first free radicals were born as a result of ultraviolet radiation. In their excitement and agitation, these free radicals formed new molecules, genetic mutations, ever different patterns like some primitive kaleidoscope until evolution came up with us. Free radicals have been part of our every cell all the way up the staircase of human development from the very first step to the pinnacle where we stand today.

The camera pulls back and back. The scene switches to a lab at the University of Michigan in 1894 and focuses on a serious young doctoral student hunched over the counter, his legs wrapped around a wooden stool, his hands busy with an experiment. Moses Gomberg had escaped to America with only the clothes on his back, one saber length ahead of the czar's soldiers. Here was a true Horatio Alger story. He went on to educate himself, become head of the chemistry department at Michigan, and the first to discover free radicals. He watched them charge around, sending off sparks of destruction, before they burned themselves out. He gave these excitable elements their name.

Time passes. The camera moves on. The calendar pages turn faster and faster (like they always do in those black-and-white movies) and then stop. The year is now 1954. And look. What do we see? A woman in a lab coat. She is Rebecca Gersman, a scientist. Rebecca and her lab partner Daniel Gilbert are doing some research on a form of blindness called retrolental fibroplasia that affected premature infants. Little bitty babies were going blind and nobody knew why. The two medical sleuths investigated and found that the air in the incubators housing the preemies had a higher concentration of oxygen than the regular air we breathe. Further experiments pointed to the culprit. It was oxygen that was making those babies blind. Rebecca went even further in her conclusions and stated that most of the damage done to living tissue was done by free radicals arising from oxygen. This was heavy stuff.

One of the most necessary things to our survival is oxygen. Oxygen is almost everywhere, a partner in every single metabolic function from breathing to digestion. Without oxygen our hearts stop pumping, our blood stops circulating, our brain stops transmitting, food doesn't get changed to energy, and we die. But the oxygen that is so critical to our survival also throws off massive amounts of free radicals that are slowly aging us, making us sick, speeding our early demise.

How does that happen? The most common free radicals are built on oxygen molecules. Why? Because oxygen molecules have two unpaired (single, as in unattached) electrons. That makes them very susceptible to free radical invasion, because free radicals have one unpaired (single, as in unattached) electron. So they get together. The result? One unpaired oxygen electron mates (a match made in cellular hell) with the one unpaired free radical electron. They become a couple. Good for them, but oxygen had two, not one, unpaired electrons. There is still one left over. The result? Back to square one. One new free radical is born. And so it goes. You see the problem? You see the cosmic dilemma here? On the one hand, oxygen is life itself; on the other, it is death. Somebody had a strange sense of humor.

MEET THE FREE RADICALS

Superoxide aka The Master Oxygen Radical

It is the first one formed. It's pretty destructive all on its own, but it also converts easily to hydrogen peroxide and produces the even more deadly hydroxyl radical.

Hydroxyl Radical

This is the most dangerous of all the free radicals. It consists of equal parts hydrogen and oxygen. And even though it lasts only a micro-fraction of a second before it self-destructs, it will attack just about any other molecule it comes into contact with in a frantic attempt for chemical stability.

Singlet Oxygen

This is a free radical formed mainly in our skin as a response to ultraviolet light.

Hydrogen Peroxide

This is a molecule that can swim right through cell walls, damaging the delicate insides and scrambling up the messages that keep us healthy. It can also form the deadly hydroxyl radical.

Lipid Peroxy Radical

This is the free radical formed when oxygen attacks the fatty acids in cell membranes. Once the attack begins, the cell membrane is damaged and cell guts begin to ooze out.

THE EXTENT OF THE DAMAGE

Free radicals spoil things. They can destroy cell membranes, the protective covering surrounding our cells. Once the membrane integrity has been breached they go even further, right into the very center of our cells, the nucleus. The nucleus is like the software in our living cellular computer. Free radicals are like a computer virus. They can seriously damage our DNA, the very plans to our entire body, and every single organ (mutagenesis). They can scramble messages. They can cause our cells to reproduce in a crazy, out-of-control fashion, become cancerous and malignant (mitogenesis). They can tap into our immune system so that we no longer can fight off various invaders. They are serious trouble. They spoil our cells, our skin, our eyes, brains, hearts, and blood vessels. And free radicals love fat. Fat gets them even more excited on a molecular level. Fat gets them to jumping and bashing into things, upsetting the natural balance and creating even more free radicals as they tear around our systems.

Free radicals have been implicated in many cancers, heart disease, cholesterol buildup, premature aging of the brain or senility, stroke, immune-system decline, vision problems and blindness, Parkinson's disease, Lou Gehrig's disease, wrinkles, liver spots, and the list goes on, and on, and on.

Free radical damage is cumulative and builds up over time and age. The older we are, the more free radical damage we sustain. The younger we are, the less free radical damage we sustain. Let's get younger.

ENTER THE GOOD GUYS, ANTIOXIDANTS

What's an antioxidant? If a free radical is a fire, an antioxidant is a bucket of water. Remember the cosmic problem? Oxygen gives both life and death? Well, there is a cosmic solution—antioxidants. An antioxidant is any substance that retards or prevents damage as a result of oxygen reactions or oxidation. Oxygen reactions throw off destructive free radicals. Antioxidants neutralize the damage done by destructive free radicals. It's a little confusing, I know. Antioxidants are not against oxygen, just the damaging garbage we call free radicals that oxygen produces. Got that?

Now understand that we don't just sit there letting free radicals do their thing. Our bodies do have a natural defense system consisting of certain enzymes. One of the most powerful internal free radical fighters is an enzyme called superoxide dismutase. We have other defenses, too. There are the internal compounds cysteine, glutathione, and D-penicillamine. We've got transferrin and the protein ceruloplasmin. All of these either prevent the formation of free radicals in the first place or mop them up wherever they appear.

But it isn't enough. Our natural defenses just aren't enough. We need help if we are not to become overrun with these destructive free radicals.

That's where dietary antioxidants come in. We have right in our own fridge, in our local grocery store enough protection to win the free radical fight. How's that? Food. That's right, food, glorious food. We can eat ourselves right out of the free radical damage zone. What a terrific solution. Food. Something we all love anyway.

So what's the catch? Sounds too good to be true? Not this time. This time it is true. Many of the diseases caused by free radicals can be uncaused by antioxidants in our food. And what food! The colors of antioxidant food! The variety! The taste! The texture! The richness! The aroma! Antioxidant foods are a feast for the eyes and medicine for the body.

MEET THE SUPERSTARS

There are four superstars in the antioxidant nutritional world—three vitamins and a mineral. Individually they are all megastars in their own right. Together, in combination, it's like the Woodstock of cellular concerts—it's as if the four Beatles got together in Strawberry Fields in

Central Park—can you imagine? Well, that's what it's like when vitamin C, vitamin E, beta-carotene, and calcium get together deep inside your very life program. It's a happening!

What do these superstars do? They do lots of good things. They patrol our cells looking for free radicals. And when they find a free radical they give it an electron, making it stable and harmless. Antioxidants can do this because they are specially designed to be able to give away their own electrons without becoming unstable or turning into free radicals themselves.

MAKING THE FOOD CONNECTION

These antioxidants—vitamin C, vitamin E, beta-carotene, and calcium—are locked deep and safe inside certain foods. And when we eat these foods, we release the antioxidants.

Eating Antioxidant-Deprived Foods

So, if you bite into a big juicy hamburger, for example, you are going to do two things. You are going to create a whole bunch of free radicals simply through the process of chewing and digestion. And you are going to create even more free radicals because when the stuff you swallowed turns into molecules, those molecules get attacked by free radicals. Any that lose an electron turn into free radicals themselves. Not so good.

Eating Antioxidant-Rich Foods

Now look what happens when you bite into a big juicy slice of cantaloupe. You are also going to do two things. You are going to create free radicals simply through the process of chewing and digestion. But you are also going to release antioxidants that destroy any free radicals that may have been created as you chewed, and are going to go on and defuse and destroy all kinds of other free radicals already there—even some of the ones from that burger. Yes!

THE DREAM TEAM

Yes, it does make sense if you think about it. Let's go back to that fantasy Beatles concert in Central Park. You've got Ringo on drums, George on lead guitar, John singing away, and Paul on bass guitar. Together you've got a group. Now that's not to say you can't have a drum solo. Sure you can. You can have one guitar playing—happens all the time. You can even have one person singing; there are walls of CDs to show that that's a highly possible and very lucrative activity. But you can also combine all those elements and come up with a group.

Antioxidants are just like that. Vitamin C is terrific on its own. It goes after those special little free radicals that love to swim and splash around in the watery parts of cells and in the special fluid between cells. Vitamin E is wonderful as a solo act, too. It goes after free radicals that attack and puncture the oily, fatty cell membranes. Beta-carotene does its own thing and so does calcium. But when you put them together, you have one powerful antioxidant, anti-aging cocktail. Vitamin C helps vitamin E be even more effective. Calcium can do a better job when it is paired up with vitamin C. Beta-carotene does its own mopping up and then helps the others. Alone they are pretty remarkable. As a group, they are awesome, restoring health, extending years, and beating back aging and premature death itself.

ANTIOXIDANTS AND LONGEVITY

Here's what we know:

- People who take vitamins, especially antioxidants, live longer than people who don't.
- Antioxidants boost aging immune systems, rejuvenating them and making them stronger and more able to fight off killer attacks from pneumonia, bacteria, viruses, and other invaders.
- Antioxidants can slow and, in some cases, even reverse the growth of cancer cells.
- Antioxidants can clean out clogged arteries, lower cholesterol levels, adjust cholesterol ratios favorably, and reduce the risk of heart attack, stroke, and hypertension.
- Antioxidants can help bones remain strong and restore lost bone tissue.

- Antioxidants can smooth wrinkles, reduce fine lines, fade age spots, and strengthen and rejuvenate collagen, the substructure of skin itself.
- Antioxidants can restore vision and keep delicate optical lenses clear and unclouded by age.
- Antioxidants can help prevent senility, diseases of the nervous system, and premature loss of brain function.
- Antioxidants protect against damage from environment pollutants like cigarette smoke, exhaust fumes, chemical sprays, and bald spots in the ozone layer.
- Antioxidants can help you shed pounds by attacking fat at its source.
- And the list goes on, and on, and on. . . .

SEARCH-AND-DESTROY MISSION

Fine, so we have all these antioxidants helping to clean up after us. So what's the problem? All we have to do is eat a couple of carrots, drink a glass of orange juice, maybe break down and have a yogurt, and we're covered. It's not quite so simple. Sure, if we make some minor adjustments in our diet we will get some minor protection. After all, a glass of skim milk with a huge burger, fries, and onion rings is better than a soda. A slice of tomato in a mayo-thick tuna salad sandwich is slightly better than no tomato at all. A piece of broccoli as a side to the twelve-ounce grilled steak and baked potato with butter is better than no broccoli at all. But it still isn't enough. It's not enough to add a token antioxidant dose and still go on gobbling down all the foods that create free radical damage in the first place. Give yourself a break today, and I don't mean what you think I mean.

We aren't doing our health, our longevity, and our weight any good unless we really make antioxidant-rich foods the bulk of our diet and all those other things an occasional, very occasional indulgence.

That's the *Fountain of Youth* secret.

There's more. It isn't just the food you eat that is aging you with massive amounts of free radicals, it's smoking, it's drinking to excess, it's sitting around on your fanny, it's weighing too much, it's living with too many stresses and no healthy outlets, it's all of these things.

See how even more important it is to flood your cells with healing, soothing, youth-enhancing antioxidants?

FRUIT AND VEGGIE DEFICIENCY

You've heard of deficiencies before? That's when you don't get enough of a certain nutrient. Well, here's a *Fountain of Youth* deficiency and one that way too many of us suffer from.

Fifty percent of Americans don't eat a single veggie or piece of fruit—ever. Ninety percent of Americans don't get their five-a-day servings of fruits and veggies.

THE RAINBOW CONNECTION

So why get so excited about fruits and veggies? Because fruits and veggies are the richest sources of antioxidants on the planet, and unless some breed of space invaders lands with a recipe for antioxidant cream pie with an antioxidant soda chaser, we are stuck with them.

Wait, there's more.

Fruits and vegetables are perfectly balanced sources of antioxidants created by nature to have just the right amount, in the right proportion to other vital nutrients, for maximum benefit and absorption.

Many fruits and vegetables contain more than one powerful antioxidant so that eating one gives you the power of two or more free radical fighters. A good example of this combo principle is broccoli (vitamin C, beta-carotene, and calcium), where you get the protection of three major antioxidant nutrients in just one food.

Fruits and vegetables are nutrient-dense. Because fruits and vegetables have such a high concentration of antioxidants, water, and fiber, there is no room left for—you guessed it—fat. So the more you eat, the less you weigh and the younger you get. Need any more reasons? I didn't think so.

RECOMMENDED DIETARY ALLOWANCES

Well, here's the beginning of the controversy. What's an RDA? Recommended Dietary Allowances are "levels of intake of essential nutrients considered . . . to be adequate to meet the known nutritional need of practically all healthy persons." The RDA for antioxidants is set in such a way as to prevent disease from a serious deficiency. However, the RDAs are not set to take into account special needs such as the fighting of infections, strenuous exercise, chronic illness, or injury. The RDA is also not set for longevity doses. So most experts agree that it is safe to get more than the RDA for the major antioxidants. In fact, most experts now recommend a longevity dose of antioxidant protection.

ANTIOXIDANT DOSAGES: A COMPARISON

	RDA	Longevity Doses
Vitamin C	60 mg	800 to 1,000 mg
Beta-carotene	50 IU	10,000 IU
Vitamin E	30 IU	400 to 800 IU
Calcium	1,000 mg	1,000 to 1,500 mg

If you get the longevity amount of antioxidants from food you can't really go wrong. However, it is very difficult to get enough vitamin E from food alone without adding massive amounts of calories to your diet. So this is one antioxidant that you may have to take in supplement form. In fact, recent Harvard studies have found that vitamin E supplements can decrease heart disease by as much as 37 percent.

THE FLAP ABOUT BETA-CAROTENE SUPPLEMENTS

In Finland, researchers doing a study gave a large group of longtime smokers beta-carotene supplements. The idea was to see if these supplements could reduce the risk of lung cancer in these folks. The results showed that there was no reduction in the risk of lung cancer, and some indication that there was more lung cancer in the group. Panic set in. The study was terminated. Other studies dealing with beta-carotene supplements were suspended. Now that the dust has settled what do we know? We know that the smokers were in a very high risk group for developing lung cancer. We know that there are hundreds and hundreds of studies showing beta-carotene in food to be a powerful and healing antioxidant fighting all kinds of diseases including cancer very successfully. We know that Nature may have included some element we still haven't figured out in food sources of beta-carotene that was left out of the synthetic version. We know that food is primo when it comes to our longevity. We know that this small ripple is no reason not to eat our carrots.

THE REST OF THE STORY

Antioxidants are true biological miracles. All we have to do is reach out and have that apple, drink that glass of fresh orange juice, have that salad, and in so doing, turn back the clock and reset the scale for a life that takes us to the max. Simple, isn't it? Wait, it gets better. Read on.

Scientists estimate that just three antioxidants—vitamins C, E, and beta-carotene—if used optimally could reduce breast cancer by 16 percent, lung cancer by 21 percent, stomach cancer by 30 percent, heart disease by 25 percent, and cataracts by 50 percent. Monetary savings of the cost of hospital care would be $1 billion for breast cancer, $3 billion for lung cancer, $30 billion for heart disease, $½ billion for stomach cancer, and $100 million for cataracts.

—Health Line, 1994

CHAPTER 5

Vitamin C:
Nature's Youth Capsule

*It is strange indeed that the more we learn about how to build
health, the less healthy Americans become.*

—ADELLE DAVIS

IT ALL STARTED IN CURAÇAO

Picture the scene. You are sitting in your seventh-grade history class, or
is it geography? It doesn't matter. You aren't paying much attention
anyway. It's a warm, lazy, spring afternoon. School is definitely not your
favorite place right this minute. It's something about explorers. Who
cares? You can barely remember the voyages of good old Christopher,
much less all those other Columbus wanna-bes. And yet the teacher
stands there, pointing at a map, droning on and on about . . .

You should have paid more attention. Because while Columbus may
have found us, Amerigo Vespucci, one of those other explorers, found
more than the new lands he had set out to discover. Amerigo sailed right
smack into a fountain of youth and didn't even know it. (See, and you
thought it was Ponce de Leon.)

It happened on just the same kind of spring afternoon that got you to
daydreaming. Only this warm afternoon was in the year 1499 on the little
Caribbean island of Curaçao. And Amerigo wasn't daydreaming, he was

busy dumping off half his crew because they were dying of scurvy—a disease that back then killed more English sailors than were lost in all the sea battles England ever fought.

A few months later, Amerigo stops off in Curaçao again and instead of the rows and rows of crosses he expects to see, he finds his crew—tanned, fit, and rum punched out. And so he named the miraculous island Curaçao, meaning "cured."

Stay with me. It wasn't until 250 years later that a British medical researcher figured out that it wasn't the rum, but the lime juice in those rum punches that cured scurvy and so on his recommendation, the British Admiralty issued every sailor on a British vessel half a lime daily with their rum allowance. Scurvy ended. The empire survived.

Some of you are way ahead of me. And that's why English sailors were called "limeys."

But even that British researcher didn't grasp the real miracle cure. And a miracle it was and continues to be. Because deep in the tart, citrusy pulp of the lime was that wonder life extender we today call vitamin C, one of the vitamin superstars in the *Fountain of Youth*.

ARE YOU IN THE VITAMIN C DEPRIVATION ZONE?

Be honest now. And take this vitamin C challenge.

1. I smoke cigarettes. (Even one or two a day count.)
2. Gotta have my bacon beside my eggs a couple of times a week.
3. I spend as much time in the sun as I can.
4. Stress? Oh, boy, I fell off the stress scale five years ago.
5. My job involves a lot of muscle. I'm not a desk person.
6. Breast cancer runs in my family.
7. Cataracts run in my family.
8. Forget fruits and vegetables and give me meat every time.
9. Vitamins are for everyone else, except me.
10. Cook? Who's got time. I'm a fast-food junkie.

I'm not going to make this easy for you. Even if you answered only one question with a YES, welcome to the vitamin C deprivation zone. This is not a fun place. The faster you get your body out of there, the longer you may live to tell your friends about it.

MEET THE MIRACLE MAKER: SECONDHAND C

So what exactly is vitamin C? Vitamin C is a water-soluble carbohydrate. That makes it a kissing cousin, biologically speaking, to glucose, known to good friends only as sugar. Great. Let's just scarf down another pint of ice cream or a candy bar and presto, chango, vitamin C. Wouldn't it be nice if it worked like that? But it doesn't. In fact, here's a little riddle just to keep you humble. What can cows, palm trees, seaweed, and most bugs do that we magnificent humans can't? Give up? Make their own vitamin C. That's right. They, along with most every living thing on this planet except for us, apes, bats, and guinea pigs—and rocks—*can* make vitamin C. Seems a little unfair, doesn't it?

While the bad news is, we can't manufacture our own vitamin C, the good news is, we *can* get enough by eating those plants and some animal products that *do* manufacture it. Let's face it, recycled vitamin C is still a powerful anti-aging weapon.

THE COLLAGEN VITAMIN

So why do we need this secondhand vitamin? What does it do? How does it keep us young? How does it keep us slender? Vitamin C's main job is to manufacture a type of cell cement called collagen. This is the stuff that keeps our complexions wrinkle-free, our hips and thighs smooth without the ugly bumps and dimples of cellulite, those plastic surgery scars healing invisibly, our smiles from developing ugly cavities, our gums sticking to our teeth, and most of all this is the stuff that helps keep our bones straight, tall, and slender.

THE WEIGHT-LOSS VITAMIN

But wait, there's more. Vitamin C also plays a role in the manufacture of serotonin—that potent brain chemical that can help you stop bingeing and lose weight. Let's not underestimate this critical function of vitamin C. We need all the serotonin we can get. In their exciting book, *The Serotonin Solution* (Fawcett Columbine, 1996), Judith Wurtman, Ph.D., and Susan Suffes explain, "We can boost serotonin simply by eating carbohydrates in the right amounts in combination with other foods. The result? Restored energy, an end to emotional overeating, and permanent weight control."

THE ANTIOXIDANT TEAM PLAYER

And now comes another very important role that this hard-working vitamin performs. Not only does it zap its own share of swimmer free radicals, those doing the crawl around the watery parts of our cells, but it also teams up with vitamin E and vitamin A—two superstars on the antioxidant dream team—and protects them from getting zapped before they can zap their own quota of free radicals. And every free radical destroyed is a cell given a whole new lease on a longer, healthier life.

A QUICK LOOK AT THE RESEARCH

Vitamin C has some very impressive credentials in the younger, thinner, and healthier forum. Check these out.

> UCLA researchers found that 300 mg of vitamin C a day added six years to a man's life and two years to a woman's life.

Reverses the Biological Clock

A British study found that vitamin C can actually reverse aging by rejuvenating white blood cells . . . giving seventy-six-year-olds the same levels as thirty-year-olds. How much vitamin C did it take? Only 120 mg of vitamin C a day—1½ cups of fresh strawberries.

Protects Skin from Ultraviolet Damage Leading to Wrinkles

Researchers at Duke University found vitamin C can make a real difference in protecting our exposed skin from the damage caused by the sun, environmental pollutants, and even cigarette smoking. The result? Fewer lines and wrinkles, less skin cancer, and a more youthful, dewy complexion.

Fights Heart Disease

Studies at the University of California found men with high levels of vitamin C in their systems were less likely to die from heart disease, especially when they had a diet rich in vitamin C and also boosted their vitamin C level with a good supplement.

Flushes Out LDL or "Bad" Cholesterol and Boosts HDL or "Good" Cholesterol

Studies at Harvard's School of Public Health have shown vitamin C fights the buildup of LDL, which can lead to coronary artery disease. Other studies at the USDA found that the levels of "good" cholesterol were highest in women getting 210 mg of calcium a day, or about the amount in a ripe cantaloupe.

Speed Recovery from Heart Attacks

A new study from India found heart attack survivors who started to eat a diet high in vitamin C had better healing of damaged heart tissue than those who didn't.

Produces Loads of Glutathione—the Sylvester Stallone of Free Radical Fighters

A study at Arizona State University found that we have more or less of the important free radical fighter glutathione, depending on how much vitamin C we get every day. How much vitamin C does it take to boost the levels of glutathione? About 500 mg does it, about the amount in three crunchy red peppers.

Vacuums Out Chunks of Fat Stuck to the Inside Walls of Our Arteries, Usually the Result of Too Many Hamburgers and Donuts

Vitamin C keeps artery walls smooth from gummy fat buildup by blocking the production of LDL. It also cleans out any LDL that is already stuck to the walls constricting blood flow.

Improves Our Immune System

According to the National Cancer Institute, vitamin C works like an antibiotic against viruses that attack and weaken our immune systems. It also triggers the production of interferon, which is one of our body's natural defenses against foreign invaders that can damage and destroy our healthy, living cells and tissue.

Reduces Our Risk of Developing Lung Problems Like Asthma, Chronic Bronchitis, and Others

New research from the U.S. Environmental Protection Agency points to the role vitamin C plays in stopping white blood cells from clumping together and sticking to the walls of blood vessels—a sign of emphysema.

Keeps Men Fertile and Protects the Delicate DNA Message in Sperm So That Babies Are Born with a Much Lower Risk of Birth Defects

Tests at the University of Texas found that infertility in men was reversed with 200 mg of vitamin C a day. There's more. The University of California at Berkeley found men with low levels of vitamin C were more likely to have defective sperm that could cause birth defects in babies. Once the men in the study went back to between 60 and 250 mg of vitamin C the DNA damage to their sperm declined within thirty days. A single orange a day could produce genetically healthier babies.

The Five-Way Cancer Fighter

As if all that weren't enough for this busy little antioxidant, it mounts a five-way attack against cancer: blocks the formation of cancer-causing elements inside our cells, blocks free radical damage to our delicate DNA threads, shuts off the cancer-starting switch certain viruses and some rogue genes like to turn on, keeps our immune function high, and last but not least, slows down the growth of unfriendly tumors.

Study after study shows people who eat a diet rich in vitamin C are also 50 percent less likely to develop some of the more deadly forms of cancer, especially breast cancer (in postmenopausal women) and cancer of the cervix.

Boosts the Benefits of Other Vitamins

A study at the Human Nutrition Research Center on Aging at Tufts University found that people who got 220 mg of vitamin C from their diet—about three oranges worth—also had the most vitamin E, another critical antioxidant and anti-aging vitamin.

Helps Us Absorb Iron

The University of Kansas Medical Center found that adding just 66 mg of vitamin C a day—about one orange—can boost the body's ability to absorb iron by a whopping 500 percent. And along with calcium, iron is the second most deficient mineral in our average diet.

The Visionary Vitamin

Vitamin C directly attacks those free radicals that cloud the lens of our eyes, causing cataracts and other premature eye conditions that impair our sight and can even leave us blind, say studies from the U.S. Department of Agriculture's Human Nutrition Center at Tufts University.

The Gum Disease Warrior

A recent study in Finland found periodontal disease is almost four times more common in people with low blood levels of vitamin C.

The Old Cold Remedy

In test tubes vitamin C has been found to be a very effective antihistamine. It not only relieves runny noses, but also attacks the germs that caused them in the first place.

THE RECOMMENDED DIETARY ALLOWANCE OF VITAMIN C

Pregnant women	80 mg
Lactating women	100 mg
Infants from birth to 6 months	35 mg
Infants from 6 months to 1 year	35 mg
Children from 1 to 10 years	45 mg
Children from 11 to 18 years	50 mg
Adults	60 mg
Heavy cigarette smokers	100 mg

NEW RESEARCH SAYS RDAS TOO LOW

Some of us don't take any vitamin C. Some of us take megadoses. Some of us are somewhere in the middle. Sometimes we take it, sometimes we don't—but we don't really know how much to take at all. Well, some of the controversy and confusion about vitamin C is closer to being resolved. A study in *The Proceedings of the National Academy of Sciences* found that the "optimal" daily intake of vitamin C was more like 200 mg and doses over 400 mg per day "have no evident value." The battle of the amounts rages on. Bottom line: you probably could use a little more Vitamin C in your diet.

TOP FOOD SOURCES OF VITAMIN C

Food	Serving in mg (All food servings are ½ cup, or 1 medium piece of fruit or vegetable, or 1 cup of juice)
Fruit	
Papaya	188
Guava	165
Black currants	101
Strawberries	85
Orange, navel	80
Kiwifruit	75
Cantaloupe	68
Mango	57
Grapefruit	47
Mandarin orange	43
Lemon	31
Honeydew melon	27
Tangerine	26
Currants	23
Casaba melon	21
Lime	20
Blackberries	15
Raspberries	15
Watermelon	15
Cranberries	13
Pineapple	12
Apricots (3 medium)	11
Banana	10
Blueberries	10
Vegetables	
Pepper, hot	109
Pepper, sweet red	95
Pepper, sweet green	64
Brussels sprouts	48
Broccoli	41
Cauliflower	36
Peas	31
Sweet potato	28

Food	Serving in mg
Vegetables	
Kale	27
Parsley	27
Collards	23
Onions	23
Potato	22
Tomato	22
Cabbage, red	20
Rutabaga	19
Asparagus	18
Beet greens	18
Cabbage, green	18
Mustard greens	18
Garden cress	17
Turnip greens	17
Cabbage, Chinese	16
Swiss chard	16
Soybeans	15
Spinach	15
Squash	15
Avocado	14
Okra	13
Lima beans	11
Dandelion greens	10
Radish	10
Juice	
Orange	124
Lemon	112
Cranberry	108
Grapefruit	94
Lime	72
Grape	60
V-8 Juice®	52
Tomato	33
Pineapple	30

VITAMIN C SUPPLEMENTS

Again we come to that Hamlet-like question: To supplement or not to supplement? Most experts agree that vitamin C is most effective when it comes from food sources because it comes in little packages with other vital anti-aging nutrients included. However, some studies show that supplements can make a difference in some forms of anti-aging protection. On the downside, if you take more than 500 mg per supplement at a time, your body won't be able to absorb the extra and it will get flushed out. Our body only takes what it needs from the vitamin C supply and flushes the rest out. But because vitamin C is a water-soluble vitamin, you need to keep replenishing the supply.

THE COMBO APPROACH

Researchers at UCLA have found that vitamin C can add years to our lives and a combination of partly diet and partly supplements may make the most sense for all of us in our busy, stressed, fast-food lives.

So, what's the answer? Eat a diet rich in vitamin C and take a supplement every day as a little extra anti-aging insurance.

A SUGGESTED ANTI-AGING DOSE

250 to 1,000 mg per day

CHAPTER 6

Vitamin E:
The Miracle Vitamin

One should eat to live, not live to eat.
—BENJAMIN FRANKLIN

PUTTING THE "E" IN S_X

It started with a rat and sex, as so many exciting discoveries do. The difference was, in this case, the rat got better and better, became a good provider of cheese, stayed home most nights, and produced the politically correct 4.7 baby rats every year. Doesn't sound like any of the rats I have known and loved. It sounds too good to be true. Sounds like a miracle, right? Right.

Welcome to the complete, unabridged story of vitamin E. This is the *It's a Wonderful Life*—the happiest of happy endings—vitamins. This is the vitamin that even some of the most conservative, I-don't-believe-in-vitamins types secretly scarf down. This is the one that even many medical journalists from the tabloids to the university presses believe in.

Vitamin E is soft, blemish-free, kissable skin; juicy, throbbing loins; slender, smooth legs; and the libido reminiscent of sweaty palms and scratchy backseats in two-door automobiles on prom night.

This is the "Oscar" of vitamins. This is the one that started with sex, made a hasty stop at fertility, a slightly longer stop at potency, and is now rushing full tilt into something better even than sex (yes, there is), and that is youth.

THE CALIFORNIA CONNECTION

It was California (where else?) in the Roaring Twenties. Cousin to the flappers, the energetic Charleston, and Prohibition, vitamin E began as a lab experiment in fertility. Scientists developed a diet high in rancid-prone fats and fed it to lab rats. (Sound familiar?) The result? Female rats stopped reproducing. When dark green leafy vegetables were added to the diet, fertility resumed. The same rancid-fat diet caused male rats' testicles to degenerate. Adding the dark green leafy vegetables restored sperm fertility and produced healthy rat babies. The researchers called this vitamin, which could turn sexual function on and off like a light switch, vitamin E. Why? Because vitamins A, B, C, and D had already been discovered and named alphabetically. E was next on the list.

Ten years later in the middle of the dark depression, vitamin E was given its "scientific" name—tocopherol from the Greek words meaning "to bear offspring."

But science hates a vacuum. It was well and good to breed bunches of sexy rats, but what about humans? And so the really interesting experiments began.

The time: 1966. The place: Columbia Medical School Hospital in New York City, a nursery filled with cranky, irritable, and very noisy babies. The problem? Their formula didn't contain any vitamin E. As soon as vitamin E was added to the bottles, the babies settled down. It had taken over forty years and thousands of rats, hamsters, and guinea pigs, but science had finally found a human condition that responded to vitamin E. And three years later, in 1969 vitamin E found itself nominated for a top ten slot on that prestigious RDA chart of must-have nutrients. And science hasn't looked back since.

To this day, vitamin E has kept its sexy image. Only now, scientists from around the world are showing that vitamin E can not only restore youthful vigor but can prolong it and more. Vitamin E has become one of the most important anti-aging vitamins we have.

COULD YOU USE A LITTLE VITAMIN E IN YOUR LIFE?

Ask yourself, Am I pretty active, running around, getting sweaty, working out? Am I a fast-food junkie? Am I one of those few remaining holdouts who huddles around a communal outdoor ashtray? Do I live with a nicotine addict? Am I a big city sophisticate? Am I about ready to buy my first pair of reading glasses? Am I still trying to convince myself those huge round things are really cute, but oversized freckles, instead of what they really are—age spots? Do I want to turn back the clock?

Be honest with yourself. If you answered YES to even one of these questions, you are a definite candidate for the miracle vitamin.

THE FAT BUSTER VITAMIN

One of the very first industrial uses for vitamin E was to retard food spoilage. Vitamin E is a fat. It works to protect the fatty parts of our cells and fights the free radicals that love to turn the fatty part of us rancid and rusty . . . like a stick of butter that has been left out on the kitchen counter too long, turning sour and dingy. If vitamin C knocks out the free radicals that attack through water like enemy submarines, then vitamin E knocks out the free radicals that crawl through the most intimate parts of our bodies. And those intimate parts of bodies, so tied to our youth and our health, are also the most vulnerable to attack by free radicals and prolonged exposure to oxygen. It is vitamin E that is credited with protecting the fragile immune cell membranes that are our first line of defense against disease, premature aging, and death; the pink insides of our artery walls that pump nutrient-rich blood to every part of our bodies and keep hearts and other vital organs working; and brain cells that regulate much of our anti-aging mechanisms.

THE "BREATH OF LONGER LIFE" ANTIOXIDANT

There is still a lot we don't know about all antioxidants, but there are some very important things we do know about vitamin E. We know that it increases the average life span of laboratory animals, helping them to reach their maximum. If it can do that for lab animals, scientists believe it can also do that for us—helping us to reach our maximum life span of 120 years.

Vitamin E is like a big umbrella spread over us, protecting our delicate cells from the damage and destruction of sunshine, oxygen, smoking, and pollution, and keeping us young inside and out.

THE KEY EXPERIMENTS

I. The Age Spot Experiment

Scientists believe that age spots are sort of rusty patches of fat, bad enough when we have to see them on the backs of our hands, but much worse where we can't see them: in our brain cells, slowing down thought function, and affecting memory and coordination. When animals were fed a diet similar to the typical standard American diet (SAD, for short), they couldn't find their way out of a simple maze. When vitamin E was added to their diets, lab animals ran through the maze with speed and accuracy. Nice.

2. The Treadmill "Bad" Breath Experiment

Researchers at the University of California knew that when athletes performed at their peak capacity they took great big deep breaths way down into the very bottom of their lungs. Those big, deep breaths flooded lung tissue with oxygen, which caused an oxidative reaction producing loads of very excited and dangerous free radicals. When they exhaled, the free radicals were measured in droplets of breath. Now here's where it gets interesting. The athletes were put on treadmills, fast treadmills. Some of them were given 1,200 IU (750 mg) of vitamin E; some were just given a placebo. After two weeks of hard running, the athletes who had taken the vitamin E were producing fewer damaging free radicals even with a strenuous exercise program. The other group was aging their lungs and flooding their entire body with 50 percent more age-producing free radicals. Which group got the better workout? Which group got younger with every step? You guessed it. The vitamin E group.

LET ME COUNT THE WAYS OR HOW VITAMIN E KEEPS US YOUNG

Slows Overall Aging

Vitamin E scrubs lipofuscin, or aging pigment, from our cells, part of the "rusting out" theory of aging, rusting brought on by exposure to oxygen and just plain day-to-day living and breathing. This lipofuscin is the rusty brown sludge that shows up as age spots on our skin, our internal organs, and most dangerously on our brain cells, scrambling important messages, speeding disease, cellular destruction, and ultimately premature death.

Keeps the "Old Ticker" from Becoming an "Old Ticker"

Studies from the University of Southern California School of Medicine found that as little as 100 IU of vitamin E daily could widen narrow, clogged arteries and shrink fatty deposits of blood vessel–blocking cholesterol. The magician vitamin E seems to change the LDL or "bad" cholesterol into HDL or "good" cholesterol.

Harvard research found that women who took between 100 and 250 IU of vitamin E daily reduced their risk of heart attack by 41 percent and stroke by 29 percent. The vitamin E ladies also had an overall decrease in mortality rates of 13 percent. Men were winners too in the same study, lowering their risk of major cardiovascular problems by 37 percent.

The stats just keep getting better. A new study found the more vitamin E women got from food sources, the higher their likelihood of not dying of heart disease—by an impressive, attention-getting 62 percent.

The Immune System Raincoat

If it's pouring free radicals out there every time we take a breath, then vitamin E coats every one of our cells with a youth-enhancing raincoat.

Research at Tufts University concluded that people who have higher levels of vitamin E in their blood have lower infection rates, less respiratory disease, and fewer colds—all indicators of a youthful, healthy, and strong immune system.

Some international experts have even gone so far as to say that the risk for not taking vitamin E may be as great as the risk of smoking when it comes to heart and blood vessel health.

Primo Cancer Fighter

Two large clinical trials support the theory that vitamin E may cut the risk of developing lung cancer and cancers of the mouth and throat by 50 percent. This is attributed directly to vitamin E's impressive credentials as an immune system booster that inhibits the growth and spread of cancer cells in the first place.

Skin Enhancer

Taken internally, vitamin E protects skin from the more visible signs of aging such as fine lines, wrinkles, and age or liver spots. Applied externally, researchers believe vitamin E can speed healing, reduce scar tissue, and protect against the development and growth of deadly skin cancers.

The Great Legs Vitamin

Hate varicose veins? Hate tired, achy legs? Hate muscle fatigue? Vitamin E to the rescue. Studies at Tufts University found that strenuous exercise releases chemicals into the muscles that make them sore, swollen, and inflamed. Vitamin E soothes away the aches and pains and even smooths out unsightly veins. So keep walking and take your vitamin E.

The Arthritis Reliever

Researchers speculate that vitamin E is quickly used up in folks with arthritis—the vitamin E rushing to the site of the swelling to fight off the free radicals. If you have arthritis, you may need more vitamin E to give you relief from the pain, swelling, and morning stiffness brought on by arthritis.

Clear Eyes

Researchers at Johns Hopkins Medical Institution found that the lower the amount of vitamin E in your diet, the greater your chances for developing cataracts.

The Dreaded Alzheimer's Disease

Some preliminary studies are beginning to point to the power of vitamin E to protect the delicate transmission sites in the brain from getting coated with aging sludge and not being able to transmit nerve messages effectively.

HOW MUCH IS ENOUGH?

Research points to the fact that most of us get enough vitamin E from our daily diet to offer us minimum protection. However, longevity experts almost without exception agree that the current RDA of 12 IU for women and 15 IU for men is not enough and we can't get enough from our diet alone. So most recommend increasing that amount to between 100 and 400 IU daily.

> Adults should take 100 to 400 IU (international units) of vitamin E a day.
> —THE ALLIANCE FOR AGING RESEARCH, WASHINGTON, D.C.

THE BEST FOOD SOURCES OF VITAMIN E

> A WORD OF CAUTION: Because vitamin E is fat soluble it is found in polyunsaturated fats such as vegetable oils. These add unwanted fat calories to the diet. The solution? A combo of dietary and supplemental vitamin E.

Food	Serving	Vitamin E (IU)
Wheat germ oil	1 tablespoon	25
Sunflower seeds	1 ounce	21
Almonds	1 ounce	11
Sunflower oil	1 tablespoon	10

Food	Serving	Vitamin E (IU)
Safflower oil	1 tablespoon	8
Asparagus	12 spears	6
Wheat germ	1 ounce	5
Margarine, soft	1 tablespoon	3
Mayo	1 tablespoon	3
Rice, brown	1 cup	3
Peanuts, dry roasted	1 ounce	3
Mango	1 medium	3
Avocado	1 medium	3
Soybean oil	1 tablespoon	2
Spinach	1 cup	1

SUPPLEMENTS

There are two types of vitamin E available in supplements. D-alpha or RRR-alpha on the label means the vitamin E is natural. Dl-alpha or all-rac-alpha means the vitamin E is synthetic. The natural form seems to be twice as well absorbed and retained as the synthetic, according to some studies.

TIP: Take your vitamin E supplement last thing at bedtime along with your calcium supplement.

WARNING: This is one vitamin you need to check with your doctor about, especially if you are taking medication to slow blood clotting.

CHAPTER 7

Beta-carotene:
The Number One Age Buster

Experience is the name everyone gives to their mistakes.
—OSCAR WILDE

THE STARS OF THE DESERT NIGHT

If you look up into the midnight sky on some clear night, you will be able to take the test, which was known in ancient Arabia over four thousand years ago as the test of the third star. There is a star called Mizar, the third star in the constellation known as the Big Dipper. Mizar has a mate, a shy, soft star called Alcor, the test star. Alcor sits at the extreme periphery of vision, so the ancients figured if you could see Alcor you passed your vision test. If you couldn't you were given carrots to eat until your night vision was restored. And restored it was. Therein lies the very first beta-carotene experiment and cure.

THE RAINBOW CONNECTION

We all know what a rainbow looks like: layers of beautiful color all joined together for one spectacular show. A rainbow wouldn't really be a rainbow if it were just orange. It wouldn't be a rainbow if it were just blue or red. A rainbow needs all the colors of the spectrum to really shine. Well, that's what happens with this really interesting vitamin.

WHAT MAKES FLAMINGOS PINK?

We've all heard of beta-carotene by now. But do we really know what it is? And have we met all its kissing cousins? Beta-carotene comes from one of those big families that just keep getting bigger, the carotenoids. Beta-carotene belongs to the branch of the family that lives in orange and dark green fruits and veggies. Lycopene, another relative, belongs to the branch that lives in tomatoes, red peppers, and other red food substances. It's the lycopene flamingos eat that eventually turns their feathers pink. The same thing happens to shrimp and lobster.

At last count there were over six hundred carotenoids and more surfacing every time scientists peek through their microscopes.

THE ADAM AND EVE OF VITAMIN A

But the remarkable thing is that current thinking believes that all these carotenoids evolved from beta-carotene. Ain't nature grand?

WHAT'S BETA-CAROTENE? WHAT'S VITAMIN A? WHAT'S THE DIFFERENCE?

Beta-carotene is what we get when we eat bright green, yellow, red, and orange fruits and vegetables. Beta-carotene is also what cows, chickens, geese, and ducks get when they eat their green grass, oats, small leafy twigs, and hay.

Now here's the magic. Once animals and humans swallow their beta-carotene meal it travels through the digestive system and when it reaches the intestine it turns into vitamin A!

That's why we can get lots of potential vitamin A from fruits and vegetables and ready-made vitamin A, also called retinol, from liver and other vital organs of animals—because their bodies already did the conversion for us.

The bottom line is that beta-carotene becomes vitamin A. But experts agree that it is best to be a vitamin A do-it-yourselfer and make our own instead of eating it secondhand, as in calves' liver or liverwurst. Why? Because the secondhand stuff comes with added fat and cholesterol—both not so very desirable.

> Fruits + Vegetables = Beta-carotene
> Beta-carotene + Digestion = Vitamin A

BETA-CAROTENE: THE STARSHIP ENTERPRISE IN A FREE RADICAL UNIVERSE

Free radicals come in all shapes and sizes to attack every kind of cell and every single component of every single cell. Beta-carotene is dispatched to seek out one very toxic and specific brand of free radical called a singlet oxygen. This Borg of the body attacks the fat or lipids, integral cell components, turns them rusty and disgusting, and finally causes them to crumble. So it's beta-carotene to the rescue.

BETA-CAROTENE AGAINST AGING

The Wrinkle Wars

Who hasn't heard of retin-A—first as a way to fight embarrassing acne, and then miraculously to beat the wrinkle clock and restore smooth, line-free, youthful skin. While this may not be one of the most life-extending values of vitamin E, it certainly has made the passing of years less stressful for a lot of people who use it. It restores self-esteem and reduces the stress of visible aging. Not bad.

Nature's Own Sunscreen

If you forget to slather on sunscreen before you go out to the beach or your job you can still get lots of protection from the inside out. Studies at Harvard have found that beta-carotene allowed patients with a severe sun sensitivity to triple their exposure to sunlight. The study showed that beta-carotene is naturally transferred to our skin and regulates the amount of damaging rays that penetrate to cause sun damage, wrinkles, and even skin cancer. Voilà, sunscreen in a carrot!

Shields Against DNA and Chromosome Damage

The single most important manual stored deep in every single one of our trillions of cells, DNA does it all, including, according to some scientists, regulating our aging clock. Free radicals like to get into that DNA and start to fool around with the main menu. Beta-carotene protects that fragile instruction book from alteration, damage, and destruction by free radicals.

Cancer Fighter Extraordinaire

What do we know about beta-carotene and cancer? Lots. But perhaps most important we know that beta-carotene is right in there at the very beginning of cancer formation, fighting to reduce its spread and reverse its damage. And it fights just about every kind of cancer free radicals can help cause.

Lung Cancer

Scientists at the University of Texas discovered that the more beta-carotene eaten, the lower the lung cancer rate. A similar study at John's Hopkins University also found that people with low levels of beta-carotene were four times more likely to develop the most deadly form of lung cancer.

That doesn't mean you can puff away between salads, though. Smokers still have a much higher rate of lung cancer—the number one cancer killer—than nonsmokers.

Breast Cancer

A study from Australia found that women with breast cancer who loaded up on beta-carotene had twelve times the survival rate of those who had low beta-carotene levels in their systems. A study from researchers in Buffalo, New York, found the same thing.

Cancer of the Cervix, Colon, and Mouth

Another group of Australian studies found that beta-carotene fought a successful battle against cancer of the cervix. A major study from the

National Cancer Institute found that a high beta-carotene intake was associated with a 32 percent reduction in cervical cancer.

Lesions in the mouth were reversed and turned back into normal cells with beta-carotene.

Colon cancer was slowed and even stopped in subjects who increased their beta-carotene intake.

A study from Harvard showed men who ate ten or more servings of tomatoes and tomato-based foods a week lowered their risk of prostate cancer by 45 percent.

Immune System Protection

Researchers at Cornell University found that subjects who had higher levels of beta-carotene in their systems showed much greater resistance to cell damage by UVA light and had a stronger immune system. Similar tests at the University of Arizona found older patients who got extra beta-carotene had more naturally occurring killer cells and T-helper cells, which protect the body from infections, viruses, and various cancers.

Heart Disease and Stroke

Recent studies show beta-carotene can reduce heart attack risk by 22 percent and the risk of stroke by 40 percent. European studies found those subjects who took in the least beta-carotene had a 260 percent higher risk of a first heart attack than those who ate their veggies regularly.

A Harvard study found that women who ate at least five beta-carotene-rich carrots a week reduced their chances of a stroke by a whopping 68 percent. Spinach eaters reduced their risk of stroke by an impressive 40 percent.

Healthy Eyes

Macular Degeneration

This is a condition that is responsible for most of the impaired vision and blindness in folks fifty-plus. A study from the Massachusetts Eye and Ear

Infirmary in Boston and other ophthalmology research centers around the country found that those with the highest intake of beta-carotene had a 43 percent lower risk for developing macular degeneration.

Cataracts

The Nurses Health Study found that beta-carotene-rich diets translate into a 39 percent lower risk of developing cataracts.

RECOMMENDED DIETARY ALLOWANCES OF VITAMIN A

Age and Status	RE
1 to 6 months	420
6 months to 3 years	400
4 years to 6 years	500
7 years to 10 years	700
Adult males	1,000
Adult females	800
Pregnant women	1,000
Nursing mothers	1,200

AVOIDING THE BETACAROTENE VS. VITAMIN A CONFUSION

Well, here we go again, just when we think we understand the permutations and finer points of the whole vitamin thing, stuff happens to complicate the issues. And here's a bit of a complication: There are no recommended daily allowances for beta-carotene, but there are some for vitamin A—the stuff that beta-carotene turns into. Great, just great! No wonder we just want to throw our hands up in the air and go out for beer, burgers, and fries. But don't. If all you want is to read a list of foods you should be eating to get maximum beta-carotene, just skip this part and go right to the list. Don't worry about the fact that there are no amounts of beta-carotene listed. Just take my word for it, those foods in my list are beta-carotene superstars—enjoy. For those of you who want a little more detail, here it comes.

IU VS. RE

And the winner is . . . before we talk about the winner, let's talk about the "fight." Because the search for the right measurements is really the best way to sort out the vitamin A vs. beta-carotene confusion.

Let's have a little review. Once upon a time, when scientists sitting on high stools in front of smelly Bunsen burners first began to measure vitamin A, they used a kind of scientific rule marked off in international units (IUs). Then, as they began the switch to computers and electron microscopes, they were able to peel back the layers of vitamin A and when they did they discovered something really interesting. You see, they had thought vitamin A was like other vitamins—pure as gold, through and through, so that if you chopped off a chunk of vitamin A you would get a smaller chunk but it would still be vitamin A.

Wrong. It turns out that vitamin A was like a rainbow vitamin—it had layers of other elements. Vitamin A was a blend of beta-carotenes, some of which came from veggies and some from cows and other animals. It's like the terrific pair of earrings I have: big loops of both gold and silver intertwined. I love those earrings because they go with whatever I'm wearing—they are a kind of no-brainer jewelry. Well, that's sort of what vitamin A is like—two vital elements intertwined from two different sources, animal and vegetable, that keep us young.

Beta-carotene—as we know it—is essentially vitamin A from plants as opposed to vitamin A from, say, liver. Great.

Now these scientists decided that they needed a way to measure vitamin A to adjust for the beta-carotene component. So they came up with a new measurement called retinol equivalents (REs). The National Academy of Sciences (the head honchos) lists the recommended daily allowance of vitamin A in REs and everyone else is playing catch-up. Until everything gets sorted out and standardized just remember this:

I RE equals 10 IU of beta-carotene from plants and 3.33 IU of vitamin A from animal foods.

Top Food Sources of Beta-carotene (Fruits and Veggies)

Apricots, dried	Mango
Apricots, fresh	Muskmelon
Beet greens	Papaya
Bok choy, fresh	Parsley
Broccoli	Peas and carrots, frozen
Cantaloupe	Peppers, red and sweet
Carrots	Pumpkin
Collard greens	Spinach
Dandelion greens	Squash, butternut
Endive	Squash, winter
Garden cress	Sweet potato
Kale	Tomato
Lettuce	Vegetable juice cocktail

Top Food Sources of Vitamin A (Animals)

Beef liver	Braunschweiger
Pork liver	(smoked liver sausage)
Chicken liver	Turkey soup
Liverwurst	Chicken soup
Turkey liver	Pâté de fois gras (goose liver)
Chicken giblets	Milk, skim

CARROTS OR PILLS? MAKING THE CHOICE

Again, the rule for most anti-aging nutrients is food sources first, supplements second as a type of insurance policy. But—and it's a very big BUT—when it comes to beta-carotene there is quite a stir among the most knowledgeable researchers in the world.

It really started in Finland just a little while ago. A group of researchers was conducting a fairly standard study to determine the effects of beta-carotene supplements on the development of cancer among longtime cigarette smokers. The results found that beta-carotene supplements had no effect and maybe even did more harm than good. These results lead to the cancellation of U.S. studies on beta-carotene supplementation. So what's the bottom line? Scientists seem to feel that health benefits may come from beta-carotene in combination with other elements found in food but not found in supplements. So, until further studies are undertaken, the best advice seems to be to eat your veggies.

BEST ANTI-AGING DOSE

The National Cancer Institute recommends at least five servings of fruit and/or vegetables every day.

CHAPTER 8

Calcium:
The Longevity Mineral

*The only way to keep your health is to eat what you don't want,
drink what you don't like, and do what you'd rather not.*

—MARK TWAIN

THE LONGEVITY MINERAL

They don't call calcium the longevity mineral for nothing. It looks like
chalk, mostly tastes like chalk, but without it we would all be a shapeless
puddle of cells. For a long time the white stuff, milk, was what we
thought of when we thought of calcium at all. And thinking about it,
how many of us can still hear our mother's voice saying, "Drink your
milk, you'll have strong bones." Well, this was one case where Mom was
right—to a point. Today, there are so many reasons for getting enough
calcium that they won't all fit into a glass of milk. But if all the reasons
were rolled into one great big reason it would be this: CALCIUM ADDS
YEARS TO YOUR LIFE. No kidding!

ARE YOU CALCIUM CHALLENGED?

So, what's your excuse? I get enough calcium from my cheeseburger. I
take a multivitamin. I'm allergic to milk. Yogurt gives me gas. I heard
that too much calcium causes kidney stones. I'm not old enough to worry

about calcium. I'm too old to worry about calcium. Wrong. Wrong. Wrong. Ask yourself this:

- Is my tummy pouchy and does it stick out no matter now many crunches I do?
- Is my hair prematurely gray?
- Am I suffering from that dieter's curse, "stuck scale syndrome"?
- Have I added a periodontist to my dental to-do list?
- Am I a breast cancer candidate?
- Is my blood pressure a tad too high?
- Am I shorter by an inch or so since my first high heels?
- Am I a woman?

If you answered YES to even one of these questions, welcome to the world of the calcium challenged. You are definitely not getting enough calcium, and like almost 90 percent of women out there, that deficiency puts you at risk for serious, life-shortening diseases. And if that doesn't get your attention, try this: A calcium deficiency can sabotage your weight loss, your posture, your energy level, your wit, and even your sexy smile.

THE 98 TO 2 FORMULA

Ninety-eight percent of the calcium in our bodies is stored in long, skinny storage units called bones. Two percent circulates throughout our bodies, carried in the bloodstream, and this little bitty amount has a big job. It keeps our hearts beating, our brains transmitting, our feet moving, our golf clubs swinging, and our blood pressure normal. If all that wasn't enough, it squashes colon cancer cells before they can do serious and deadly damage. Calcium is so important that our own bodies don't trust that we are going to get enough every day. That's why every little bit of extra calcium is stored, hoarded away for that rainy bone day. How much do we need every day? Seven hundred milligrams—just about what you would find in a couple of glasses of skim milk and half a cheese sandwich. If you don't swallow that amount every day, it comes out of your storage. If you take too much out of your storage too often, pretty soon the storage tank—or bones—crumble and fall apart. So give your body a break and take the calcium challenge.

CALCIUM GETS AN "A" FOR ANTIOXIDANT

Every little bit of calcium is important. But our bones may not be able to absorb and store calcium to the max because of the interference of free radicals. These little devils "steal" the oxygen we need for calcium to be properly absorbed. This may cause damage to our skeleton and speed the onset of osteoporosis and other premature aging diseases. Now calcium comes to the rescue! As an antioxidant mineral calcium blocks the oxygen starvation leading to diminished bone mass, protects cell membranes from destruction by free radicals, and creates a calcium "thermometer" to regulate the level of calcium in blood and bones.

CALCIUM VS. "THE BIGGIES"

Osteoporosis

This is a crippler and a killer. Starting around the age of thirty, all of us are in the very early stages of potential osteoporosis. If we don't do anything about it, gradually it gets worse and worse, until twenty years later we sneeze, lift a bag of groceries, or try for that overhead shot and break a neck bone, vertebra, or a hip. And broken bones are a reality for over 50 percent of women over the age of fifty. Once that bone breaks, your life will never be the same. Twenty-five percent of you with a hip fracture won't be able to walk a year later. But that's still better than another 25 percent who will have died as a result of complications. So much for a long and healthy life. Not possible without calcium.

> More women die of osteoporosis than of breast cancer, cancer of the cervix, and cancer of the uterus combined.

Heart Disease

Want to go from fat, clogged arteries to slick, smooth arteries? One of the best ways to get there is with calcium. Calcium actually lowers the "bad" cholesterol that clogs arteries by as much as 11 percent and raises the "good" cholesterol, reducing the risk for heart disease—that number one life shortener—by 20 percent.

> Researchers recommend a low-fat diet and at least 1,000 mg of calcium per day from a combination of food and supplements.

Blood Pressure

Not only does calcium seem to be able to lower blood pressure that is resistant to a sodium-restricted diet, but scientists have found that it can also prevent high blood pressure from building up in the first place. Getting 1,200 mg of calcium per day reduces your risk for developing high blood pressure by 12 percent—25 percent if you are under forty according to a massive study by the National Center for Health Statistics.

Colon Cancer

Calcium has been shown to protect against the development of colon cancer, ranked number two in the cancer family, and may even reverse already present cancer cells in the colon.

> The University of California at San Diego found that folks who drank 2½ glasses of milk a day had one-third the rate of colon cancer as those who didn't.

The Fat Fighter

The good news is that calcium may block the amount of saturated fat we actually absorb. Researchers at Oklahoma State University think that calcium may stick to fat molecules and flush them out of our system before they have a chance to settle into stubborn pounds, flab, and folds. The danger here is that the calcium gets flushed too.

THE NATIONAL INSTITUTES OF HEALTH
NEW CALCIUM RECOMMENDATIONS

Age and Status	Mg per Day
Infants from birth to 6 months	400
Infants from 6 months to 1 year	600
Children from 1 to 5 years	800
Children from 6 to 10 years	800 to 1,200
Adolescents from 11 to 24 years	1,200 to 1,500
Pregnant adolescents	2,000
Pregnant women	1,200 to 1,500
Premenopausal women 25 to 50	1,000
Postmenopausal women on estrogen	1,000
Postmenopausal women not on estrogen	1,500
Men 25 to 65	1,000
Men 65 plus	1,500

NOW FOR THE BAD NEWS: CALCIUM ROBBERS

Before you get too excited and start popping calcium supplements and slugging down big frosty glasses of milk, you need to pay a little attention to calcium blockers—substances that can "steal" half or more of the calcium you think is going straight to your bones to keep you young and strong.

Calcium Robber #1: Salt

Think of what happens to a patch of ice when you toss some salt on it in the dead of winter. A few minutes later it is riddled with holes. Guess what? The same thing happens to our bones when we sprinkle them with too much salt. There's more. Salt is a pushy bully. Not only does it erode the calcium already in our bones, but it blocks new calcium from entering bone storage.

The AMERICAN JOURNAL OF CLINICAL NUTRITION reports that 2,600 mg of sodium can wipe out 891 mg of calcium—that's practically your whole day's worth.

Calcium Robber #2: Caffeine

The bad news here is that the amount of caffeine you take in may be proportional to the amount of calcium you lose. The good news is that researchers now feel that three cups of coffee per day are not a calcium risk, especially if you add a little skim milk to each cup. And coffee isn't the only caffeine culprit. Watch out for iced tea, hot tea, hot chocolate, cocoa, colas, and some medications.

Calcium Robber #3: Fat

Fat can combine with calcium and convert it to a chunky form that can't be absorbed, so our body throws it out with the rest of our trash. The result? We get fatter and our bones get thinner—not a good combination.

Calcium Robber #4: Protein

I know what you're going to say: We need lots of protein. Well, if you said that, you would be half right. We do need protein, but we don't need lots of it. To give you an idea, women need about the amount of protein every day that's in a couple of cups of milk—and guys don't need very much more. In fact, if you have a chicken breast for dinner and a cup of milk on your morning cereal, you've reached your protein goal for the day. See any burgers there? Any cheese puffs? Any sixteen-ounce sirloins? Nope. Preliminary research is finding that too much protein causes our kidneys to work overtime, flushing out all the protein sludge and with it much of the calcium. So when it comes to protein, less protein may mean more calcium.

Calcium Robber #5: Smoking

Besides the fact that women who smoke enter the menopause zone a few years younger and with 5 to 10 percent less bone mass, smoking creates a cloud of free radicals that destroys delicate bone tissue, attacks calcium stored in bones, and leaves us very vulnerable to a mass of premature aging problems.

> The Osteoporosis Center at the Hospital for Special Surgery in New York says that smokers have twice as much a chance of getting a back fracture as nonsmokers.

Calcium Robber #6: Alcohol

Here is where a little alcohol may be good for your bones, raising estrogen levels, protecting your heart, and lowering your blood pressure. But too much—more than a glass of wine a day—is deadly, sucking calcium out of bones and weakening them fast.

> A Harvard University study showed that regularly drinking a substantial number of alcoholic beverages increases the likelihood of breaking both a hip and an arm.

Other Calcium Robbers to Watch

Too much fiber can block calcium from being absorbed. The solution? Don't cut down on your fiber intake—increase your calcium intake.

Oxalic acid and phytic acid found in some veggies like spinach, green beans, and beet and turnip greens can wipe out the high calcium content of these wonderful veggies. The solution? Sprinkle a little vinegar or lemon juice on top before you eat them. The acid helps release the calcium and makes it easier to absorb.

Medications like some antacids, cholesterol regulators, and thyroid and arthritis medications may block the absorption of calcium. Check with your doctor and ask about a calcium-boosting regimen to protect your bones.

TOP FOOD SOURCES OF CALCIUM

Dairy Food	Mg Calcium
Yogurt, plain, nonfat, 1 cup	452
Yogurt, plain, low-fat, 1 cup	415
Cheese, Parmesan, 1 ounce	355
Yogurt, fruit-flavored, low-fat, 1 cup	314
Milk, skim, 1 cup	302
Cheese, Romano, 1 ounce	301
Milk, 1%, 1 cup	300
Milk, 2%, 1 cup	297
Buttermilk, 1 cup	285
Milk, chocolate, 2%, 1 cup	284
Cheese, Swiss, 1 ounce	272
Cheese, Cheddar, 1 ounce	204
Cheese, mozzarella, part skim, 1 ounce	183
Ice milk, ½ cup	137
Ice cream, ½ cup	118
Yogurt, frozen, ½ cup	89

Protein Food	Mg Calcium
Tofu, ½ cup with calcium sulphate	434
Sardines, canned with bones, 4 ounces	272
Salmon, canned with bones, 4 ounces	242
Beans, lima, 1 cup cooked	144
Tofu, ½ cup without calcium sulphate	130
Perch, baked, 3 ounces	117
Almonds, ¼ cup	94
Beans, Great Northern, ½ cup	61
Beans, kidney, 1 cup	50

Fruits and Veggies	Mg Calcium
Spinach, fresh, ½ cup cooked	122
Turnip greens, fresh, ½ cup cooked	99
Kale, frozen, ½ cup cooked	90

Broccoli, fresh, ½ cup cooked	89
Okra, fresh, ½ cup cooked	88
Beet greens, fresh, ½ cup cooked	82
Bok choy, fresh, ½ cup cooked	79
Mustard greens, frozen, ½ cup cooked	75
Collard greens, fresh, ½ cup cooked	74
Frozen mixed veggies, 1 cup cooked	59
Orange, 1 medium	52
Tomato juice, 1 cup	22
Pear, 1 medium	19
Carrot, 1 medium	19
Raisins, ¼ cup	18

Grains	Mg Calcium
Waffle, 7 inches diameter	179
Pancakes, 2, 4 inches diameter each	72
Bread stuffing, 1 cup cooked	64
Rice, brown, 1 cup cooked	63
Hamburger roll	54
Baking powder biscuit	47
Corn tortilla	42
White bread, 1 slice	32
Bagel	29

TO SUPPLEMENT OR NOT TO SUPPLEMENT?

If you are struggling with this question, don't. Experts agree that when it comes to anti-aging protection and enhancement from calcium both food choices and supplements should be part of the program.

BE SUPPLEMENT SMART

Read the label. Talk to your health care professional. And add supplements to your calcium-rich diet. Here are some guidelines:

- Calcium carbonate contains the most elemental calcium (40 percent) and is the most widely used.

- Calcium citrate comes in second on elemental calcium (24 percent) and is the most easily absorbed, causing the fewest tummy troubles.
- Calcium lactate comes in third (13 percent) on elemental calcium and contains lactate, which helps in absorption, but which is not a good idea if you are lactose intolerant.

HOW TO TAKE YOUR SUPPLEMENTS

To get the most benefit from your calcium supplements you should take them in divided doses—no more than 600 mg at a time between meals with orange juice, milk, or yogurt to help in the absorption. Make sure you take your last calcium supplement just before bedtime because most of the calcium seeps out of our bones while we sleep.

DO THE VINEGAR TEST

Drop your calcium supplement into a glass of vinegar. Wait 30 minutes. If it hasn't dissolved, switch brands. You need to get calcium supplements that dissolve fast for maximum benefit.

A SUGGESTED ANTI-AGING DOSE

1,200 mg to 1,500 mg per day

PART THREE

FOUNTAIN OF YOUTH
ANTI-AGING WEIGHT-LOSS
PROGRAM

CHAPTER 9

Getting Younger, Getting Thinner, Getting Ready

It takes about ten years to get used to how old you are.
ANONYMOUS

YOU'RE IN THE MAJORITY

According to one of those cute little charts scattered through the pages of *USA Today*, two-thirds of us want to lose weight. We want to lose somewhere between five and fifty pounds. And that's a good thing, too, because just about two-thirds of us *need* to lose weight. We are toting around way too much fat. Well, here is where you can put down that load.

COME FLY WITH ME

Find a couple of suitcases. Go on, I know you've got them stashed in the attic, or basement, or in the back of that closet you've been meaning to clean out for months. Now I want you to throw some stuff into them. What you pack doesn't matter. You don't have to be neat. This is just going to be an experiment. Keep packing until the two cases together weigh between twenty and thirty pounds. That's about ten to fifteen pounds per case. Got that?

Now pick up those two suitcases and walk around with them. Go into the kitchen. Tuck one under your arm and try opening the fridge without dropping it. Now take them upstairs. Bring them back down. Sit down and balance them in your lap while you check the weather on TV. Get up with them. Walk into the bedroom. Hold them tight. Walk into the bathroom. Come on, just a little while longer. Keep doing this for about ten minutes or so. Are you getting a little tired yet? Wasn't it harder to get up those stairs? Aren't you a little more winded than you would be just walking around your own house normally? Doesn't your pulse race a bit? Perhaps you've even gotten a little hot and sweaty.

Okay, good. Drop those suitcases. Now take that same trip through your house. How do you feel? Light. Like you could fly. Your pulse has slowed down. You've stopped sweating. You are moving with more speed and agility. You even feel happier. Those tight lines around your mouth from gritting your teeth have smoothed out.

Hold on to that feeling because that's what it feels like to lose twenty or thirty pounds. That's what it feels like to be lighter. That's what it feels like to be younger. That's how you're going to feel in a few short weeks. Great, isn't it?

WHY THIS PROGRAM WORKS WHEN OTHERS HAVE FAILED YOU

1. This is not a diet.

This is a nutrient-dense antioxidant-rich food plan designed to slow the aging of your body at the cellular or molecular level. One of the most exciting by-products of this revolutionary anti-aging program is dramatic weight loss.

2. This is not a deprivation program.

There is so much food to eat, your problem may be finishing it. Unlike other programs that tightly and rigidly restrict portions, quantities, and foods, this program loads you up with six meals a day, a wide variety of foods, and lots of the foods you love to eat—the ones that leave you feeling full and satisfied. This is not a deprivation program. On the contrary, it is an abundance program.

3. This is a naturally low-fat program.

Because the emphasis is on foods that are antioxidant dense, the same foods that are so filled with goodness, there is no room for excess fat. You will naturally be eliminating fat without even realizing it or missing it.

4. This is a healthy, safe, and balanced program.

This is not a program that focuses on a single food. It isn't protein heavy. It doesn't force you to count grams, calories, or servings. This program isn't hard work. It is easy. And the foods you will enjoy are the foods you love anyway.

5. This is a high energy program.

Because you will be flooding your body at the cellular level with restorative and rejuvenating antioxidants, your energy level will rise. You won't feel sluggish or fatigued. These high energy levels will keep you inspired and motivated.

6. Foods on this program are filling.

Forget juice diets. Forget liquid protein. Forget grapefruits. Forget dry snacks. These meals, all six of them, are filling. They are packed with satisfying carbohydrates and fiber, which give you not just a sensation of satisfaction, but really satisfy you. When you add the antioxidant nutrients, your body will not be starved for nutrition but sated. It will be easier for you to stay on this program as a result.

7. Snack attacks are covered.

Satisfying meals are provided that cover the most vulnerable times of the day: the midmorning, late afternoon, and bedtime periods when so many of us experience a real food low. Extra antioxidants available at those critical times make sure that you don't ever get too hungry and slip.

8. Generous portions are the norm.

You won't have to look at a tiny little helping lost and forlorn in the middle of a huge dinner plate. You won't have to "cheat" and put your allocated meals on little side or salad plates. You are going to be eating very, very generous portions. It will take you a long time to eat each meal. You will *feel* full. You will *be* full.

9. This is an inexpensive program.

You don't have to buy any special foods. You don't have to go to any meetings. You don't have to spend time and money on complicated preparations. You don't have to shop for exotic and hard-to-find food. All you have to do is go to your favorite grocery store and follow the handy shopping lists. Watch your food bill get slashed when you fill your shopping cart with antioxidants and leave out the empty calories.

10. This program works fast.

    You won't have long to wait. You will feel results fast. You will see results fast. And your results will last a lifetime.

WHAT THE PROGRAM IS ALL ABOUT

It's all about you. The *Fountain of Youth Anti-Aging Weight-Loss Program* is all about you. Simple. It's about you looking younger. It's about you feeling younger. It's about you getting younger. It's about you finally losing that weight and keeping it off. It's about you having the energy, vitality, and sheer love of life you had years ago. It's about you getting healthier. That's what this program is all about—you.

HOW FAST WILL YOU LOSE THE WEIGHT AND THE YEARS?

I designed this as a ninety-day program. All the research I've done points to the fact that it takes at least ninety days to make any significant changes in our weight and health. So don't roll your eyes and think it's too long. Let's get real. We all know you can't lose fifteen pounds in a day and a half no matter what some of the ads say. And we also know, don't we, because we've tried it, that even if through some biological and metabolic miracle we did lose fifteen pounds on Tuesday, it would all come back on Wednesday plus five extra pounds on Thursday. Right?

    As far as how fast you will lose—I don't know. We are all different. But here is a chart that shows you how much and how fast I lost. Pay attention. There were some very frustrating plateaus—actually deserts— in there. But I got through them and so will you.

Day 1	168 (My starting weight)
Day 2	166
Day 3	165
Day 4	164½ (That's the water gone.)
Day 5	165
Day 6	165½
Day 7	166 (STOP. This is the WRONG direction.)
Day 8	166 (This is the stupidest idea I ever had.)
Day 9	165½
Day 10	165½

Day 11	165
Day 12	164¼ (Haven't I been here before?)
Day 13	164½
Day 14	163½ (Terrific! 4½ pounds in two weeks.)
Day 15	164 (It was dumb to celebrate with a pizza.)
Day 16	163½ (Okay, I can make up for it.)
Day 17	163½
Day 18	163½ (How long must I be punished for that pizza?)
Day 19	163
Day 20	162
Day 21	162½ (Only 1 pound lost this week. Too bad.)
Day 22	162
Day 23	160½ (Wow! Now we're talking.)
Day 24	161
Day 25	161½ (I'm getting really dizzy with this up and down stuff.)
Day 26	160½
Day 27	160½
Day 28	160
Day 29	161
Day 30	161½ (Well, there's the first thirty days and I've only lost 6½ pounds. This is going to take me forever.)
Day 31	160½
Day 32	159½ (I can't believe it. I'm actually in the 150s.)
Day 33	158 (Yes! Now we're cookin'.)
Day 34	158½
Day 35	158½
Day 36	157 (I knew I shouldn't have had that glass of wine or those corn chips, or that guacamole, or that chocolate chip cookie. Why? Why did I have that glass of wine?)
Day 37	157 (Okay, maybe the damage isn't so bad.)
Day 38	158½ (That's right, punish me. One little glass of wine. It's over. I should have known. I'll just give it another day.)
Day 39	159 (I give up. No. I'll give up tomorrow.)
Day 40	158 (I'm not giving up today. I can do this.)
Day 41	158
Day 42	157½ (I'm not going to get all excited just yet in case it doesn't last.)
Day 43	157
Day 44	156½ (It's going to be okay.)
Day 45	156½

Day 46	156½ (The good news is, I'm stuck in the 150s not the 160s.)
Day 47	156
Day 48	155 (Thank you. Thank you. Thank you.)
Day 49	155½ (This doesn't scare me anymore.)
Day 50	155½
Day 51	155
Day 52	154½
Day 53	154
Day 54	154½
Day 55	154
Day 56	154½ (I'm getting seasick again.)
Day 57	154
Day 58	154
Day 59	154
Day 60	154 (Maybe this is what I'm supposed to weigh?)
Day 61	153 (I'm two-thirds of the way through and I've lost 15 pounds. That's great. And I feel pretty good, too. In fact, I just bought a new outfit—two sizes smaller than usual.)
Day 62	152½
Day 63	152½
Day 64	152 (I got my hair done today and the hairdresser noticed I looked thinner.)
Day 65	151½
Day 66	151½
Day 67	150½ (Please let me get below 150. Please. I'll never ask for anything again.)
Day 68	151 (Sorry I asked.)
Day 69	150½
Day 70	150
Day 71	150 (I thought today would be the day I broke through into the 140s. Oh, well, don't get discouraged. There's plenty of time left.)
Day 72	148½ (YES!!!)
Day 73	148 (I did it. I'm ahead of schedule.)
Day 74	149 (Better not stop yet.)
Day 75	149
Day 76	149½ (I can't believe this.)
Day 77	149½
Day 78	149

Day 79	149
Day 80	148½
Day 81	148½
Day 82	148½
Day 83	148 (Okay, if I can stay here for at least three days in a row, I'll know I made it.)
Day 84	148
Day 85	149½ (NO!!!)
Day 86	149
Day 87	148
Day 88	148
Day 89	147½
Day 90	148 (Congratulations, Edita, you did it!!!!)

HOW YOUR WEIGHT WILL CHANGE

You are going to lose weight. You are going to lose fat. You are going to shift things around so that you fit in your clothes better. You'll stop jiggling. You will feel lighter, more airy. You will rediscover belts. And the fat you lose will not just be the ugly, puckered stuff you can see on the outside, but the sticky, yellowish blobs floating around on the inside, too.

HOW YOUR HEALTH WILL CHANGE

It will change for the better. Here's what is likely to happen to you. It did to me.

√   Your blood pressure should go down.
√   Your resting pulse should get slower.
√   Your cholesterol level should go down.
√   Your cholesterol ratio should improve.
√   You should sleep better.
√   You should have more energy.
√   Your mood and general outlook on life should perk up.
√   Your immune system should be stronger.
√   Your skin should look clearer and smoother.
√   Your bones should get stronger.

√   Your joints should stop feeling stiff and achy.
√   Your night vision should improve.
√   And the list goes on and on and on . . .

WHAT KEEPS YOUR HEART HEALTHY: WEIGHT LOSS OR EXERCISE?

Researchers at the University of Maryland compared weight loss to aerobic exercise and found that weight loss was the winner. Weight loss lowered "bad" cholesterol and raised "good" cholesterol, and lowered blood glucose, insulin, and blood pressure. But don't give up that walking.

HOW YOU WILL GET YOUNGER WITH EVERY BITE

When your health improves and your weight gets down to normal levels, you are doing two very important anti-aging things for yourself:

1. You are delaying the onset of aging, aging diseases, helplessness, loss of dignity, and fear of death.
2. You are giving yourself back lost years. You are going backwards to when you were five, seven, ten, or more years younger.

Vanity Benefits Short Term

- You'll get your figure back better than ever.
- You will look and feel years younger.
- You will be the envy of all your friends, both the ones who like you and the ones who can't stand you.
- Your spouse will be proud of you.
- No spouse? You might even get a date at the end of this program.
- Your kids, grandkids (if you admit to any), nieces, nephews, and other assorted relatives will be shocked and surprised at the wonderful new you. (It's almost worth it just for that alone.)
- Your grocery bill will go down, and you'll have more money for those new outfits you'll need.

- Your skin will glow, fine lines will fade, and your eyes will sparkle with life and youth.
- You'll like looking in mirrors again.
- You will start thinking about taking up new activities, making new friends, taking new trips—and you'll actually do all of it!

Long-Term Benefits
- Hours, days, weeks, months, and years more of life can be yours through this program.
- Aches and pains should fade away and disappear.
- Your risk of serious health problems, like cancer, heart disease, stroke, diabetes, osteoporosis, arthritis, and high blood pressure, will be significantly reduced.
- Your ability to slow the advance and possibly even reverse the progress of chronic diseases you may already have will improve.
- Your immune system will be stronger.
- Your body will be flooded with healing antioxidants, every cell bathed in a nutrient-rich formula that will simply make you healthier.

GETTING PSYCHED, GETTING STARTED

Are you ready? This is it. Just a few more practical items to take care of and you are ready to start my *Fountain of Youth: The Anti-Aging Weight-Loss Program*. I know you can hardly wait. But please be patient just a little longer and read these very important instructions. We are going to be together for at least the next ninety days. I want nothing more than for you to get younger and thinner with every bite, every meal, every day. And I know you do, too. So, make sure you follow these next instructions and assemble everything you will need ahead of time. Make sure you fill out the personal weight and age chart. Make sure that you have tested your own body age so that you have something to really compare your progress against when you have completed the formal part of the program. Don't skip anything now. These few last-minute items can save you frustration and time. So, let's both make sure you get off to a good start so that you can finish a success!

Fountain of Youth:
The Anti-Aging Weight-Loss Program Guidelines

1. You won't be hungry.
2. You will eat six meals a day, including snacks.
3. My three special *Fountain of Youth* recipes are specially designed to be tasty and attractive and to give you the maximum youth and skinny nutritional benefits.
4. Every single day has been designed so that you have just the right number of calories. There's no need for you to count a thing.
5. Every single day has been designed so that you have loads of anti-aging nutrients to make you younger and melt off those aging pounds.
6. Each day has been very carefully designed, so please don't invent your own menu until you have completed the entire ninety-day program. You can get more creative when you are on the maintenance program.
7. Try to eat everything for every day.
8. It's okay not to eat the individual meals in order. If you feel like having dinner for lunch, go ahead. Just don't skip anything and don't add anything of your own.

WARNING: If you are allergic to something in this program, don't eat it. You can skip foods that disagree with you. Just don't add anything of your own to make up the difference.

EDITA'S "MUST DO DAILY"

You must walk for 30 minutes every day. Try walking for 15 minutes away from your home or office, then walk back.

    This is nonnegotiable.

It's almost time. I know you have read everything up to this point and are eager to get started. You can hardly wait to start getting thinner and younger with every single bite. There are just a few more last-minute items to cover that will save you lots of time so that you can really devote yourself to this exciting new program.

Preview the Program

Flip through and take a good look at the actual *Fountain of Youth: The Anti-Aging Weight-Loss Program.* Previewing the program will give you some idea of the wonderful foods you will be eating, the large number of satisfying meals you can expect, the variety of different items available to you, the ease of preparation—no slaving over a stove here. Make sure you understand the program and that you are starting it as a truly well-informed participant. Get familiar with it. Get comfortable with it.

Go Shopping Now If You Have To

Now for the food part. You will be very pleasantly surprised at how much food you will be able to eat every day. Because there is so much to eat, you need to stock up and not run out halfway through the week. I've made it very easy for you with prewritten shopping lists. Take a few minutes and look over the shopping lists that are coming up and make sure you have everything you need in stock. If you don't, go to the store. You need to have at least one week's worth of anti-aging foods on hand. Nothing can sabotage your efforts faster than not being prepared properly and finding yourself out of key anti-aging ingredients.

Fill Out Your Starting Point Data Sheets

You're not really ready to start until you jot down the measurements and readings you have taken that reflect your true biological age on the data sheets at the very beginning of the program before you start. You will find similar data sheets at the end so that you can really see how remarkable your success for your first ninety days really was. Once you see how much younger, slimmer, and healthier you have become in a short time, you will be truly ready to continue the *Fountain of Youth: The Anti-Aging Weight-Loss Program* for life.

Get Naked!

There is just one more thing I want you to do: Get naked! Go ahead, take off every single stitch of clothing you are wearing now (if you are at work, it's a good idea to wait until you get home and into the privacy of your own bathroom), and take a good long look. Turn around. Check out those lumps, rolls, and bumps. Look at yourself front, back, and sideways—both sides.

And then say good-bye. Say good-bye to the flab. Say so long to the fat. Wave to the love handles. Shake that behind *arrivederci*. Bid a fond adieu to those puffy boobs, those chubby thighs, those wiggly-wobbly arms. Grin at those lines and wrinkles. Kiss them all good-bye. Because in just a few short weeks you are going to get naked again, only this time you are going to say hello to the slender, tight, youthful, healthy new body you have eaten your way into one delicious, nutritious, anti-aging mouthful at a time!

Personal Data Sheet. The Beginning: Start Date _____

These tests are all in Chapter 3. I strongly urge you to take them before you begin the program. The critical concept behind this program is that you will not only get thinner, but you will get younger as well. So let's find out just how old you are before you start.

Test 1: The Skin Pinch Bio-Test
Body Age Result _____
Test 2: The Resting Heart Rate Bio-Test
Body Age Result _____
Test 3: The Big Blur or Visual Acuity Bio-Test
Body Age Result _____
Test 4: The Systolic Blood Pressure Bio-Test
Body Age Result _____
Test 5: The Cholesterol Bio-Test
Body Age Result _____
Test 6: The Weight Bio-Test
Body Age Result _____
Final Body Age (Add up all the ages for all the tests and divide the result by 6 to find your final body age) _____

Now, just for fun, take the following measurements in inches. You'll be surprised in ninety days when you compare your final results to these.

Bust _____

Waist _____

Hips _____

Upper Right Arm_____   Upper Left Arm_____

Upper Right Thigh_____   Upper Left Thigh_____

Personal Data Sheet. The End: End Date _____

Test 1: The Skin Pinch Bio-Test
Body Age Result _____

Test 2: The Resting Heart Rate Bio-Test
Body Age Result _____

Test 3: The Big Blur or Visual Acuity Bio-Test
Body Age Result _____

Test 4: The Systolic Blood Pressure Bio-Test
Body Age Result _____

Test 5: The Cholesterol Bio-Test
Body Age Result _____

Test 6: The Weight Bio-Test
Body Age Result _____

Final Body Age (Add up all the ages for all the tests and divide the result by 6 to find your final body age) _____

Now, just for fun, take these measurements in inches. Then compare these results with the ones you recorded at the start.

Bust _____

Waist _____

Hips _____

Upper Right Arm_____   Upper Left Arm_____

Upper Right Thigh_____   Upper Left Thigh_____

SEARCH-AND-DESTROY MISSION: AGING FOODS

This is the fun part. If you live alone, take all these foods and either throw them out or take them to a church or shelter. If you live with a spouse or kids, weed through as many of these aging foods as you can. The rest should be stored in one or two cupboards in your pantry, far enough away so that you won't be tempted.

Ready? Got those garbage bags out? Got those cartons ready? Get rid of these enemies of youth and slenderness.

Ice cream
Whole milk
Sour cream
Cream cheese
Cheeses that aren't nonfat or low-fat
Assorted crackers
Frozen desserts
Frozen veggies in prepared sauces
Cookies, cakes, donuts, sweet treats
Snack foods (including potato chips, pretzels, ready-bagged popcorn)
Butter, margarine, and other spreads
Beer, wine, alcoholic beverages, sodas
Canned fruits in heavy syrup
Candy
Assorted salad dressings that aren't nonfat, including mayonnaise
Assorted condiments, such as barbecue sauce, ketchup, and cream-based
    mustards
Cream soups

GETTING YOUR KITCHEN READY FOR FOUNTAIN OF YOUTH COOKING

You will be surprised how easy cooking and cleaning up will be on this program. Foods are kept close to their natural and healthy state so cooking is fast. You will have loads more time to get to some of those fun projects you always wanted to start. You'll have lots more time to go for that walk and look through that catalogue for some great new clothes. You'll see.

1. Nonstick skillets and pans, including a wok
2. Microwave-safe containers
3. Plastic storage containers in assorted sizes
4. Garlic press

5. Kitchen shears
6. A set of sharp knives
7. Egg separator (optional)
8. Steamer basket
9. Broiler pan
10. Juicer
11. Colander
12. Salad spinner (optional)
13. Blender
14. Food processor

NOW, LET'S GO SHOPPING

I have organized two seven-day shopping lists to make it easy for you to keep supplies of anti-aging and weight-loss foods on hand. Many of the items are staples, which you already may have in your kitchen. You don't have to buy those; just make sure you have enough so you don't run out. If you do buy staple items from the first shopping list, you don't have to buy them again until you run out. Even though items are repeated, staples will last you a very long time.

After the second week you will have a good idea of the supplies you need. Just take a few minutes and read through the food lists for days 15 through 22 and days 23 through 30 and make up your own shopping lists based on the requirements.

Store breads in the freezer and use as needed.
Buy fruits and veggies fresh and often.
If you have a choice, always choose nonfat.
Buy small sizes and quantities.

**Shopping List Day 1
Through Day 7**

Total® Whole Grain Cereal
Raisin bran cereal
English muffins
Pancake mix, blueberry
Rice cakes, any flavor
Bagels, 2
Oatmeal (instant is fine)
Whole wheat bread, low-fat or
    low-calorie
Popcorn for air popping
Pita bread
Skim milk
Yogurt, low-fat or nonfat, fruit
    flavored
Yogurt, low-fat or nonfat, plain
Salad dressing, nonfat, assorted
    flavors
Parmesan cheese, grated
Cheddar cheese, low-fat
Mozzarella cheese, low-fat
Cream cheese, low-fat
Eggs
Spaghetti
Spaghetti sauce, tomato, low-fat
All-fruit preserves, any flavor
Tomato soup, 1 can
Vegetable juice, 1 can
Salsa
Brown sugar
Maple syrup
Coffee
Tea
Bottled water (tap water is fine)
Chicken breast, skinned and
    boned, 1
Turkey, white meat, 4 ounces

Flounder fillet, 4 ounces
Smoked salmon, 1 small package
Tuna, canned, packed in water
Oranges, 2
Grapefruit, 1
Cantaloupe, 3
Tomatoes, 3
Apple, 1
Bermuda onion, 1
Baking potatoes, 4
Carrots, 1 package
Celery, 1 bunch
Sweet potato, 1
Brussels sprouts, 1 small package
Strawberries, 1 pint

**Shopping List Day 8
Through Day 14**

Bagels, 2
English muffins
Oatmeal
Whole wheat bread, low-fat or
    low-calorie
Rice cakes
Raisin bran cereal
Total® Whole Grain Cereal
Popcorn for air popping
Pita bread
Raisin bread
Spaghetti
Coffee
Tea
Bottled water (tap water is fine)
Vegetable juice
Raisins
All-fruit preserves, any flavor
Brown sugar
Maple syrup

Honey

Spaghetti sauce, low-fat

Yogurt, low-fat or nonfat, fruit
flavored

Yogurt, low-fat or nonfat, plain

Skim milk

Eggs

Parmesan cheese, grated

Swiss cheese, low-fat or nonfat

Cheddar cheese, low-fat or nonfat

Cream cheese, low-fat or nonfat

Salad dressing, nonfat, assorted
flavors

Salsa

Chicken noodle soup

Vegetable soup

Red peppers, 2

Sweet potato, 1

Baking potatoes, 3

Orange, 1

Tomatoes, 2

Cucumber, 1

Bermuda onion, 1

Apple, 1

Carrots, 1 package

Celery, 1 bunch

Tuna, packed in water

Flounder fillet, 4 ounces

Turkey breast, 8 ounces

Chicken breast, 1

Salmon fillet or steak, 4 ounces

Hamburger patty, 1

THREE SPECIAL FOUNTAIN OF YOUTH RECIPES

I have developed three very special recipes for you. You will find them on
the menu almost every day because they are an integral part of my
Fountain of Youth program.

Let me tell you about them.

EDITA'S FOUNTAIN OF YOUTH SALAD

This is not just another boring "old" salad with your basic iceberg lettuce,
pale tomatoes, and wrinkled slice of onion all drowned in some disgusting oily dressing. Not a chance. This is a very special anti-aging
blend of Nature's most antioxidant-dense foods. This salad can turn back
the clock and give each one of your tired old cells a rejuvenating boost of
energy and vitality. Each one of the ingredients has been carefully chosen
because each one is a powerhouse of nutrition. Every single ingredient in
this salad contains not just one youth nutrient, but two and sometimes
even three or more!

Check it out for yourself and you'll see why this special salad is such a
vital part of my weight-loss and anti-aging program.

EDITA'S <u>FOUNTAIN OF YOUTH</u> SALAD

This is one of the most wonderful dishes in the program. This salad, which you can make ahead of time and store in your fridge, is filled with wonderful anti-aging nutrients. You can snack on it anytime.

1 serving = 6 cups
½ serving = 3 cups

1 head of romaine lettuce, torn into bite-size pieces
3 bunches of green onions, sliced fine
3 bunches of parsley, chopped fine
3 tomatoes, quartered
1 bunch of celery, chopped fine
1 sweet red pepper, seeded and chopped
1 sweet green pepper, seeded and chopped
1 10-ounce package salad spinach, chopped

In a large bowl, combine all the ingredients. Measure out 6 cups and place in a plastic bag. Continue filling plastic bags with 6 cups of the salad mixture until it is all used up.

Store in your fridge for an instant anti-aging salad treat.

EDITA'S <u>FOUNTAIN OF YOUTH</u> VEGGIES

Here is another staple dish of the *Fountain of Youth: The Anti-Aging Weight-Loss Program* to make ahead of time and munch on whenever you like. This combo of veggies is wonderful raw or steamed. It has been carefully selected to give you maximum anti-aging nutrients.

Makes 1 serving

1 cup broccoli, washed and cut into florets
1 cup carrots, either the mini ones or regular carrots chopped into chunks
1 cup cauliflower, washed and cut into florets
1 cup brussels sprouts, washed and sliced

Combine all the ingredients and store in a plastic bag in the fridge until ready to use.

EDITA'S FOUNTAIN OF YOUTH FRUIT SALAD

The wonderful anti-aging and weight-loss benefits of fruit are captured in this fruit combination. Make it up ahead of time and store it in an airtight container in your fridge. You'll get younger and thinner with every bite.

Makes 10 servings

1 cantaloupe, peeled, seeded, and cut into chunks
1 pound strawberries, washed, hulled, and quartered
1 pound seedless grapes, washed and pulled off vines
2 oranges, peeled and cut into chunks
1 grapefruit, peeled and cut into chunks

Combine all the ingredients in a large plastic bowl. Cover tightly and store in the fridge until needed.

Shopping List for Edita's *Fountain of Youth* Recipes

1 head of romaine lettuce
3 bunches of green onions
3 bunches of parsley
3 tomatoes
1 bunch of celery
1 sweet red pepper
1 sweet green pepper
1 10-ounce package salad spinach
1 bunch of broccoli

1 package of carrots
1 head of cauliflower
1 package of brussels sprouts
1 cantaloupe
1 pound strawberries
1 pound red or green seedless grapes
2 oranges
1 grapefruit

My *Fountain of Youth* Contract

I,_____, contract with myself, to devote the next ninety days to getting thinner, younger, and healthier. I will faithfully observe the food days outlined in this program. I will not be impatient, understanding that it took me a long time to get the way I am now. I will focus on my health. I will focus on my body. I will focus on my needs.

Signed this day _____

_____
Signature

You Have Questions? I Have Some Answers

1. What if I'm allergic to something on the program?
Simple. Don't eat it. Don't substitute. Just skip the food you are allergic to and move on.

2. What if I don't like something on the program?
Eating food you liked got you to where you are right now. You have two choices. Eat it anyway or don't.

3. Do I have to eat everything that's set out each day?
Try.

4. Do I have to eat the meals in order?
No. You can have dinner for breakfast. You can have lunch for dinner. You can switch your snacks around. Eat what is convenient.

5. What treats can I have on this program?
You will get younger and thinner. How's that for a couple of terrific treats? But that's not all. There's more. You will enjoy pancakes and French toast. There are bagels and cream cheese and even smoked salmon. There are hamburgers. There's chicken and stuffing. This is not a denial program. There are loads of foods that you love.

6. What about calories?

They are already figured out for every day. You will be averaging about 1,200 to 1,500 calories every day. Don't panic. I know that sounds like a little bit—but the foods you will be enjoying are so nutrient dense that you can eat lots of them without caloric penalties. You won't be hungry.

7. What about fat? Do I have to count fat grams?

You don't because I already did. This is an extremely low-fat diet. A given day averages about 15 percent fat from total calories. That's half of the American Heart Association recommendation and way below the average 40 percent-plus of the typical American diet. Again, don't worry. You will be so busy eating, you won't miss the fat.

8. What condiments can I use?

If you have read the daily food selections you know that nonfat yogurt mixed with salsa is a frequent topping for baked potatoes and vegetables. Nonfat salad dressing is allowed. I also allow Butter Buds®, mustard, lemon juice, and nonfat mayonnaise (don't go crazy with it), but the foods themselves are so incredibly delicious that your taste buds will soon hate the taste of fat and crave the taste of lean.

9. Can I use salt?

No. Again, it's one of those things you won't miss after a while. Experiment with spices, herbs, and juices.

10. What if I cheat?

Just don't get the guilts—and get right back on the program. Give yourself a break. All this is going to take some time. After all you didn't get this way in ninety days—the least you can do is give yourself ninety days to try something new.

11. My family won't like this plan.

So? Your boss won't like it either. Your mother might not like it. All you need to concern yourself with is whether or not *you* like it. This is about you and the rest of your life, no one else's.

12. I can't drink that much water.

Yes, you can.

13. **Can I substitute foods from the shopping list for food on the program?**

Sure. But only after you have completed the ninety-day program.

14. **Why are there snacks at bedtime?**

Because I like a snack at bedtime.

15. **What if I have to eat out?**

There is chicken, lettuce, tomatoes, baked potatoes, and fresh fruit in practically every restaurant in this country.

16. **Is this a program I should include my spouse in?**

Only if you don't want to outlive him. Of course you should include your spouse, your kids, your parents—even the family dog would benefit from this program. If you don't tell them they are on a special program they might not even notice.

17. **What happens if I want to lose less than twenty pounds?**

Lucky you. Now, how much younger do you want to get? I recommend ninety days. That's how long it takes to break old habits. Try to stick with it. Trust me, you won't wither away to nothing.

18. **What happens if I want to lose more than twenty pounds?**

Welcome to the real world with the rest of us. What you do then is when you get to the end of Day 90, turn back to the front of the program and start all over again with Day 1. Keep going till you get your weight where you want it, and then go on the maintenance program.

19. **I don't have time to walk.**

Find some. End of discussion.

20. **Does this really work?**

Just look at the cover of this book. You are looking at a fifty-year-old former chubby. Now ask that question again.

On Your Mark
Get Set
Go for It!

CHAPTER 10

Fountain of Youth:
The Anti-Aging Weight-Loss Program
Day by Day

DAY 1

Breakfast
1 cup Total® cereal
½ cup skim milk
1 orange
Black coffee or tea and 8 ounces
water

Morning Snack
½ cantaloupe

Lunch
2 slices low-calorie whole wheat
bread
1 tomato
1 ounce skim milk mozzarella
cheese
3 cups Edita's Fountain of Youth
Salad
2 tablespoons nonfat salad
dressing

Black coffee or tea and 8 ounces
water

Afternoon Snack
1 cup nonfat fruit yogurt
½ cantaloupe

Dinner
4 ounces skinless chicken breast,
baked, broiled, or grilled
4 cups Edita's Fountain of Youth
Veggies, steamed
3 cups Edita's Fountain of Youth
Salad
2 tablespoons nonfat salad
dressing
Black coffee or tea and 8 ounces
water

Bedtime Snack
2 slices low-calorie whole wheat
bread

1 teaspoon all-fruit preserves
1 cup skim milk

DAY 2

Breakfast
1 bagel
1 teaspoon all-fruit preserves
Black coffee or tea and 8 ounces
    water

Morning Snack
1 cup Edita's Fountain of Youth
    Fruit Salad

Lunch
4 ounces tuna (packed in water)
3 cups Edita's Fountain of Youth
    Salad
2 tablespoons nonfat salad
    dressing
Black coffee or tea and 8 ounces
    water

Afternoon Snack
1 cup Edita's Fountain of Youth
    Fruit Salad

Dinner
1 baked potato
4 cups Edita's Fountain of Youth
    Veggies, steamed
4 cups Edita's Fountain of Youth
    Salad
1 cup nonfat plain yogurt
½ cup salsa
Black coffee or tea and 8 ounces
    water

Bedtime Snack
2 slices low-calorie whole wheat
    bread
1 teaspoon all-fruit preserves
1 cup skim milk

DAY 3

Breakfast
1 English muffin
2 teaspoons all-fruit preserves
1 orange
Black coffee or tea and 8 ounces
    water

Morning Snack
1 cup carrots
1 cup celery
½ cup plain nonfat yogurt
¼ cup salsa

Lunch
2 slices low-calorie whole wheat
    bread
1 egg
3 cups Edita's Fountain of Youth
    Salad
2 tablespoons nonfat salad
    dressing
Black coffee or tea and 8 ounces
    water

Afternoon Snack
1 cup Edita's Fountain of Youth
    Fruit Salad
1 fig cookie

Dinner

4 ounces white meat turkey, baked, broiled, or grilled
1 cup brussels sprouts, steamed
1 sweet potato, baked
3 cups Edita's Fountain of Youth Salad
2 tablespoons nonfat salad dressing
Black coffee or tea and 8 ounces water

Bedtime Snack

2 rice cakes
1 teaspoon honey
1 cup skim milk

DAY 4

Breakfast

1 cup oatmeal
1 tablespoon brown sugar
1 grapefruit
Black coffee or tea and 8 ounces water

Morning Snack

½ cantaloupe

Lunch

1 rice cake
1 cup tomato soup made with water
3 cups Edita's Fountain of Youth Salad
2 tablespoons nonfat salad dressing
Black coffee or tea and 8 ounces water

Afternoon Snack

1 cup air-popped popcorn
1 teaspoon grated Parmesan cheese

Dinner

4 ounces flounder, broiled
1 baked potato
3 cups Edita's Fountain of Youth Salad
2 tablespoons nonfat salad dressing
Black coffee or tea and 8 ounces water

Bedtime Snack

1 cup raisin bran
½ cup skim milk

DAY 5

Breakfast

2 slices low-calorie whole wheat toast
2 teaspoons all-fruit preserves
Black coffee or tea and 8 ounces water

Morning Snack

1 cup vegetable juice
2 rice cakes

Lunch

1 bagel
1 teaspoon cream cheese
2 ounces smoked salmon
1 tomato, sliced
½ Bermuda onion, sliced

Black coffee or tea and 8 ounces
   water

Afternoon Snack
1 cup nonfat fruit yogurt

Dinner
1 baked potato
4 cups Edita's Fountain of Youth
   Veggies, steamed
½ cup salsa
3 cups Edita's Fountain of Youth
   Salad
2 tablespoons nonfat salad
   dressing
Black coffee or tea and 8 ounces
   water

Bedtime Snack
1 cup Edita's Fountain of Youth
   Fruit Salad

DAY 6

Breakfast
1 cup strawberries
1 cup nonfat fruit yogurt
½ cup raisin bran
Black coffee or tea and 8 ounces
   water

Morning Snack
2 rice cakes
2 teaspoons all-fruit preserves

Lunch
2 slices low-calorie whole wheat
   bread

1 ounce low-fat Cheddar cheese
3 cups Edita's Fountain of Youth
   Salad
2 tablespoons nonfat salad
   dressing
Black coffee or tea and 8 ounces
   water

Afternoon Snack
½ cantaloupe

Dinner
1 cup cooked spaghetti
½ cup spaghetti sauce
1 teaspoon grated Parmesan
   cheese
3 cups Edita's Fountain of Youth
   Salad
2 tablespoons nonfat salad
   dressing
Black coffee or tea and 8 ounces
   water

Bedtime Snack
1 slice low-calorie whole wheat
   bread
1 teaspoon all-fruit preserves
1 cup skim milk

DAY 7

Breakfast
3 blueberry pancakes
2 tablespoons maple syrup
Black coffee or tea and 8 ounces
   water

Morning Snack
1 apple
½ cup carrots
½ cup celery

Lunch
1 pita bread
1 tomato, sliced
¼ Bermuda onion, sliced
3 cups Edita's Fountain of Youth
   Salad
2 tablespoons nonfat salad
   dressing
Black coffee or tea and 8 ounces
   water

Afternoon Snack
1 cup air-popped popcorn
1 teaspoon grated Parmesan
   cheese

Dinner
4 cups Edita's Fountain of Youth
   Veggies, steamed
1 baked potato
3 cups Edita's Fountain of Youth
   Salad
2 tablespoons nonfat salad
   dressing
Black coffee or tea and 8 ounces
   water

Bedtime Snack
½ cantaloupe

DAY 8

Breakfast
1 bagel
1 teaspoon all-fruit preserves
Black coffee or tea and 8 ounces
   water

Morning Snack
1 cup nonfat fruit yogurt

Lunch
4 ounces tuna (packed in water)
2 slices low-calorie whole wheat
   bread
3 cups Edita's Fountain of Youth
   Salad
2 tablespoons nonfat salad
   dressing
Black coffee or tea and 8 ounces
   water

Afternoon Snack
1 rice cake
1 ounce low-fat Swiss cheese
1 sweet red pepper

Dinner
4 ounces skinless chicken breast,
   baked, broiled, or grilled
1 sweet potato, baked
4 cups Edita's Fountain of Youth
   Veggies, steamed
Black coffee or tea and 8 ounces
   water

Bedtime Snack
1 cup raisin bran
½ cup skim milk

DAY 9

Breakfast
1 English muffin
1 cup nonfat fruit yogurt
Black coffee or tea and 8 ounces
    water

Morning Snack
1 cup Edita's Fountain of Youth
    Fruit Salad

Lunch
1 pita bread
1 tomato, sliced
½ cucumber, sliced
¼ Bermuda onion, sliced
¼ cup salsa
Black coffee or tea and 8 ounces
    water

Afternoon Snack
1 cup air-popped popcorn
1 teaspoon grated Parmesan
    cheese

Dinner
1 baked potato
1 ounce low-fat Cheddar cheese
3 cups Edita's Fountain of Youth
    Salad
4 cups Edita's Fountain of Youth
    Veggies, steamed
2 tablespoons nonfat salad
    dressing
Black coffee or tea and 8 ounces
    water

Bedtime Snack
1 cup Edita's Fountain of Youth
    Fruit Salad

DAY 10

Breakfast
1 cup oatmeal
1 tablespoon brown sugar
1 orange
Black coffee or tea and 8 ounces
    water

Morning Snack
1 cup nonfat fruit yogurt

Lunch
1 cup chicken noodle soup
3 cups Edita's Fountain of Youth
    Salad
2 tablespoons nonfat salad
    dressing
Black coffee or tea and 8 ounces
    water

Afternoon Snack
1 slice low-calorie whole wheat
    bread
1 tomato

Dinner
4 ounces salmon
1 baked potato
4 cups Edita's Fountain of Youth
    Veggies
2 tablespoons nonfat salad
    dressing

Black coffee or tea and 8 ounces
water

Bedtime Snack
1 cup Edita's Fountain of Youth
Fruit Salad

Day 11

Breakfast
1 cup Total® cereal
½ cup skim milk
1 cup Edita's Fountain of Youth
Fruit Salad
Black coffee or tea and 8 ounces
water

Morning Snack
1 cup nonfat fruit yogurt

Lunch
4 ounces skinless turkey breast
2 slices low-calorie whole wheat
bread
1 tomato
Black coffee or tea and 8 ounces
water

Afternoon Snack
1 apple
1 cup carrots
1 cup celery

Dinner
1 cup spaghetti
½ cup spaghetti sauce
1 teaspoon grated Parmesan
cheese

3 cups Edita's Fountain of Youth
Salad
2 tablespoons nonfat salad
dressing
Black coffee or tea and 8 ounces
water

Bedtime Snack
1 slice low-calorie whole wheat
bread
1 teaspoon all-fruit preserves

Day 12

Breakfast
1 cup nonfat fruit yogurt
½ cup raisin bran
1 cup Edita's Fountain of Youth
Fruit Salad
Black coffee or tea and 8 ounces
water

Morning Snack
1 cup carrots
1 cup celery
1 red pepper

Lunch
1 cup vegetable soup
2 rice cakes
1 teaspoon cream cheese
Black coffee or tea and 8 ounces
water

Afternoon Snack
1 cup Edita's Fountain of Youth
Fruit Salad

Dinner

4 ounces skinless turkey breast,
  broiled, baked, or grilled
4 cups Edita's Fountain of Youth
  Veggies, steamed
3 cups Edita's Fountain of Youth
  Salad
2 tablespoons nonfat salad
  dressing
Black coffee or tea and 8 ounces
  water

Bedtime Snack

1 slice low-calorie whole wheat
  bread
1 teaspoon honey

DAY 13

Breakfast

2 slices French toast
2 tablespoons maple syrup
Black coffee or tea and 8 ounces
  water

Morning Snack

1 cup Edita's Fountain of Youth
  Fruit Salad

Lunch

4 ounces tuna (packed in water)
3 cups Edita's Fountain of Youth
  Salad
2 tablespoons nonfat salad
  dressing
Black coffee or tea and 8 ounces
  water

Afternoon Snack

1 cup air-popped popcorn
¼ cup raisins

Dinner

4 ounces flounder, baked or
  broiled
4 cups Edita's Fountain of Youth
  Veggies, steamed
3 cups Edita's Fountain of Youth
  Salad
2 tablespoons nonfat salad
  dressing
Black coffee or tea and 8 ounces
  water

Bedtime Snack

2 slices low-calorie whole wheat
  bread
2 teaspoons all-fruit preserves

DAY 14

Breakfast

1 bagel
1 egg
1 sliced tomato
Black coffee or tea and 8 ounces
  water

Morning Snack

1 cup vegetable juice
½ cup carrots
½ cup celery

Lunch

1 hamburger patty, grilled

3 cups Edita's Fountain of Youth
   Salad
2 tablespoons nonfat salad
   dressing
Black coffee or tea and 8 ounces
   water

Afternoon Snack
1 cup Edita's Fountain of Youth
   Fruit Salad

Dinner
4 cups Edita's Fountain of Youth
   Veggies, steamed
1 baked potato
¼ cup salsa
Black coffee or tea and 8 ounces
   water

Bedtime Snack
1 cup skim milk
1 slice raisin bread

Day 15

Breakfast
1 cup Total® cereal
½ cup skim milk
1 grapefruit
Black coffee or tea and 8 ounces
   water

Morning Snack
2 rice cakes
2 teaspoons all-fruit preserves

Lunch
1 pita bread
1 tomato
¼ cup lettuce
1 ounce low-fat Cheddar cheese
Black coffee or tea and 8 ounces
   water

Afternoon Snack
½ cup nonfat fruit yogurt
½ cup raisin bran

Dinner
4 ounces canned salmon
4 cups Edita's Fountain of Youth
   Veggies, steamed
3 cups Edita's Fountain of Youth
   Salad
1 baked potato
2 tablespoons nonfat salad
   dressing
Black coffee or tea and 8 ounces
   water

Bedtime Snack
1 cup Edita's Fountain of Youth
   Fruit Salad
1 fig cookie

Day 16

Breakfast
2 slices low-calorie whole wheat
   bread
1 tomato
1 ounce low-fat Cheddar cheese
Black coffee or tea and 8 ounces
   water

Morning Snack
1 cup Edita's Fountain of Youth
    Fruit Salad

Lunch
4 ounces tuna (packed in water)
1 tomato
½ cup plain nonfat yogurt
¼ cup salsa
Black coffee or tea and 8 ounces
    water

Afternoon Snack
3 cups Edita's Fountain of Youth
    Salad
1 slice low-calorie whole wheat
    bread
2 tablespoons nonfat salad
    dressing

Dinner
1 sweet potato, baked
4 ounces chicken breast, broiled,
    baked, or grilled
3 cups Edita's Fountain of Youth
    Salad
2 tablespoons nonfat salad
    dressing
Black coffee or tea and 8 ounces
    water

Bedtime Snack
1 cup Total® cereal
½ cup skim milk

DAY 17

Breakfast
1 cup oatmeal
2 teaspoons maple syrup

1 orange
Black coffee or tea and 8 ounces
    water

Morning Snack
1 cup nonfat fruit yogurt
½ cup raisin bran

Lunch
2 slices low-calorie whole wheat
    bread
2 ounces sliced turkey breast
3 cups Edita's Fountain of Youth
    Salad
2 tablespoons nonfat salad
    dressing
Black coffee or tea and 8 ounces
    water

Afternoon Snack
2 rice cakes
2 teaspoons all-fruit preserves

Dinner
1 baked potato
1 teaspoon grated Parmesan
    cheese
4 cups Edita's Fountain of Youth
    Veggies, steamed
½ cup nonfat plain yogurt
¼ cup salsa
Black coffee or tea and 8 ounces
    water

Bedtime Snack
1 cup Edita's Fountain of Youth
    Fruit Salad
1 slice raisin bread

Day 18

Breakfast
1 English muffin
2 teaspoons all-fruit preserves
1 cup Edita's Fountain of Youth
   Fruit Salad
Black coffee or tea and 8 ounces
   water

Morning Snack
½ cup carrots
½ cup red and green peppers
1 rice cake

Lunch
1 egg
2 slices low-calorie whole wheat
   bread
1 tomato
½ Bermuda onion
2 tablespoons nonfat salad
   dressing
Black coffee or tea and 8 ounces
   water

Afternoon Snack
1 cup air-popped popcorn
1 teaspoon grated Parmesan
   cheese

Dinner
1 cup spaghetti
½ cup tomato sauce
3 cups Edita's Fountain of Youth
   Salad
2 tablespoons nonfat salad
   dressing

Black coffee or tea and 8 ounces
   water

Bedtime Snack
1 cup Edita's Fountain of Youth
   Fruit Salad

Day 19

Breakfast
1 bagel
2 teaspoons cream cheese
2 teaspoons all-fruit preserves
Black coffee or tea and 8 ounces
   water

Morning Snack
1 cup Edita's Fountain of Youth
   Fruit Salad
1 cup nonfat fruit yogurt

Lunch
3 cups Edita's Fountain of Youth
   Salad
4 ounces canned salmon
2 tablespoons nonfat salad
   dressing
Black coffee or tea and 8 ounces
   water

Afternoon Snack
1 cup Edita's Fountain of Youth
   Fruit Salad

Dinner
1 baked potato
1 teaspoon grated Parmesan
   cheese

3 cups Edita's Fountain of Youth
  Salad
2 tablespoons nonfat salad
  dressing
4 cups Edita's Fountain of Youth
  Veggies, steamed
½ cup nonfat plain yogurt
¼ cup salsa
Black coffee or tea and 8 ounces
  water

Bedtime Snack
2 slices low-calorie whole wheat
  bread
2 tablespoons all-fruit preserves

DAY 20

Breakfast
1 cup Total® cereal
½ cup skim milk
1 grapefruit
Black coffee or tea and 8 ounces
  water

Morning Snack
2 rice cakes
2 teaspoons all-fruit preserves

Lunch
2 slices low-calorie whole wheat
  bread
1 tomato
½ Bermuda onion
3 cups Edita's Fountain of Youth
  Salad
2 tablespoons nonfat salad
  dressing

Black coffee or tea and 8 ounces
  water

Afternoon Snack
1 apple
1 ounce low-fat Cheddar cheese

Dinner
3 cups Edita's Fountain of Youth
  Salad
2 tablespoons nonfat salad
  dressing
4 cups Edita's Fountain of Youth
  Veggies, steamed
½ cup nonfat plain yogurt
¼ cup salsa
1 baked potato
Black coffee or tea and 8 ounces
  water

Bedtime Snack
1 cup Edita's Fountain of Youth
  Fruit Salad
1 slice raisin bread

DAY 21

Breakfast
3 buttermilk pancakes
2 tablespoons maple syrup
Black coffee or tea and 8 ounces
  water

Morning Snack
½ cup carrots
½ cup celery

Lunch

1 baked potato
½ cup nonfat plain yogurt
¼ cup salsa
Black coffee or tea and 8 ounces
water

Afternoon Snack

1 cup air-popped popcorn
1 teaspoon grated Parmesan
cheese

Dinner

1 ground beef patty, broiled or
grilled
3 cups Edita's Fountain of Youth
Salad
2 tablespoons nonfat salad
dressing
4 cups Edita's Fountain of Youth
Veggies, steamed
Black coffee or tea and 8 ounces
water

Bedtime Snack

1 apple
1 fig cookie

Day 22

Breakfast

1 cup nonfat fruit yogurt
½ cup Total® cereal
Black coffee or tea and 8 ounces
water

Morning Snack

1 cup Edita's Fountain of Youth
Fruit Salad

Lunch

2 slices low-calorie whole wheat
bread
1 ounce low-fat Cheddar cheese
1 tomato
½ Bermuda onion
2 tablespoons nonfat salad
dressing
Black coffee or tea and 8 ounces
water

Afternoon Snack

½ cantaloupe

Dinner

4 ounces skinless chicken breast,
baked, broiled, or grilled
1 cup stuffing
3 cups Edita's Fountain of Youth
Salad
2 tablespoons nonfat salad
dressing
Black coffee or tea and 8 ounces
water

Bedtime Snack

1 bagel
2 teaspoons all-fruit preserves

Day 23

Breakfast

½ cantaloupe
2 slices low-calorie whole wheat
bread
2 teaspoons all-fruit preserves
Black coffee or tea and 8 ounces
water

Morning Snack
1 grapefruit
1 cup nonfat fruit yogurt

Lunch
1 egg
3 cups Edita's Fountain of Youth
 Salad
2 tablespoons nonfat salad
 dressing
Black coffee or tea and 8 ounces
 water

Afternoon Snack
2 rice cakes
2 teaspoons all-fruit preserves

Dinner
4 cups Edita's Fountain of Youth
 Veggies, steamed
3 cups Edita's Fountain of Youth
 Salad
2 tablespoons nonfat salad
 dressing
1 baked potato
Black coffee or tea and 8 ounces
 water

Bedtime Snack
1 cup Edita's Fountain of Youth
 Fruit Salad

DAY 24

Breakfast
1 cup oatmeal
1 tablespoon brown sugar

1 grapefruit
Black coffee or tea and 8 ounces
 water

Morning Snack
½ cantaloupe

Lunch
1 rice cake
1 cup tomato soup made with
 water
3 cups Edita's Fountain of Youth
 Salad
2 tablespoons nonfat salad
 dressing
Black coffee or tea and 8 ounces
 water

Afternoon Snack
1 cup air-popped popcorn
1 teaspoon grated Parmesan
 cheese

Dinner
4 ounces flounder, broiled, baked,
 or grilled
1 baked potato
3 cups Edita's Fountain of Youth
 Salad
2 tablespoons nonfat salad
 dressing
Black coffee or tea and 8 ounces
 water

Bedtime Snack
1 cup Total® cereal
½ cup skim milk

DAY 25

Breakfast
2 slices French toast
2 tablespoons maple syrup
Black coffee or tea and 8 ounces
   water

Morning Snack
1 cup nonfat fruit yogurt

Lunch
1 cup vegetable soup
3 cups Edita's Fountain of Youth
   Salad
2 tablespoons nonfat salad
   dressing
Black coffee or tea and 8 ounces
   water

Afternoon Snack
1 slice low-calorie whole wheat
   bread
1 tomato

Dinner
4 ounces salmon, broiled, baked,
   or poached
1 baked potato
4 cups Edita's Fountain of Youth
   Veggies, steamed
2 tablespoons nonfat salad
   dressing
Black coffee or tea and 8 ounces
   water

Bedtime Snack
1 cup Edita's Fountain of Youth
   Fruit Salad

DAY 26

Breakfast
1 English muffin
1 cup nonfat fruit yogurt
Black coffee or tea and 8 ounces
   water

Morning Snack
1 cup Edita's Fountain of Youth
   Fruit Salad

Lunch
1 pita bread
1 tomato
½ cucumber
¼ Bermuda onion
¼ cup salsa
Black coffee or tea and 8 ounces
   water

Afternoon Snack
1 apple
1 cup carrots
1 cup celery

Dinner
1 cup spaghetti
½ cup spaghetti sauce
1 teaspoon grated Parmesan
   cheese
3 cups Edita's Fountain of Youth
   Salad
2 tablespoons nonfat salad
   dressing
Black coffee or tea and 8 ounces
   water

Bedtime Snack
1 slice low-calorie whole wheat
   bread
1 teaspoon all-fruit preserves

DAY 27

Breakfast
1 slice low-calorie whole wheat
   bread
1 teaspoon all-fruit preserves
1 cup Edita's Fountain of Youth
   Fruit Salad
Black coffee or tea and 8 ounces
   water

Morning Snack
1 cup vegetable juice
2 rice cakes

Lunch
1 bagel
1 tablespoon cream cheese
2 ounces smoked salmon
1 tomato
½ Bermuda onion, sliced
Black coffee or tea and 8 ounces
   water

Afternoon Snack
1 cup nonfat fruit yogurt

Dinner
4 cups Edita's Fountain of Youth
   Veggies, steamed
½ cup plain nonfat yogurt
¼ cup salsa

3 cups Edita's Fountain of Youth
   Salad
2 tablespoons nonfat salad
   dressing
Black coffee or tea and 8 ounces
   water

Bedtime Snack
1 cup Edita's Fountain of Youth
   Fruit Salad
1 fig cookie

DAY 28

Breakfast
1 cup strawberries
1 cup nonfat fruit yogurt
½ cup raisin bran
Black coffee or tea and 8 ounces
   water

Morning Snack
2 rice cakes
2 teaspoons all-fruit preserves

Lunch
2 slices low-calorie whole wheat
   bread
1 ounce low-fat Cheddar cheese
3 cups Edita's Fountain of Youth
   Salad
2 tablespoons nonfat salad
   dressing
Black coffee or tea and 8 ounces
   water

Afternoon Snack
½ cantaloupe

Dinner
4 ounces flounder, baked, broiled, or grilled
1 sweet potato, baked
3 cups Edita's Fountain of Youth Salad
2 tablespoons nonfat salad dressing
Black coffee or tea and 8 ounces water

Bedtime Snack
1 slice low-calorie whole wheat bread
1 teaspoon all-fruit preserves
1 cup skim milk

Day 29

Breakfast
1 bagel
1 teaspoon all-fruit preserves
Black coffee or tea and 8 ounces water

Morning Snack
½ cantaloupe

Lunch
4 ounces tuna (packed in water)
3 cups Edita's Fountain of Youth Salad
2 tablespoons nonfat salad dressing

Black coffee or tea and 8 ounces water

Afternoon Snack
1 cup Edita's Fountain of Youth Fruit Salad

Dinner
1 baked potato
4 cups Edita's Fountain of Youth Veggies, steamed
1 cup plain yogurt
½ cup salsa
3 cups Edita's Fountain of Youth Salad
2 tablespoons nonfat salad dressing
Black coffee or tea and 8 ounces water

Bedtime Snack
1 slice low-calorie whole wheat bread
1 teaspoon honey
1 cup skim milk

Day 30

Breakfast
3 blueberry pancakes
2 tablespoons maple syrup
Black coffee or tea and 8 ounces water

Morning Snack
1 apple
2 rice cakes

Lunch

1 pita bread
1 tomato
¼ Bermuda onion
3 cups Edita's Fountain of Youth Salad
2 tablespoons nonfat salad dressing
Black coffee or tea and 8 ounces water

Afternoon Snack

1 cup air-popped popcorn
1 teaspoon grated Parmesan cheese

Dinner

4 ounces skinless chicken breast, broiled or baked
1 baked potato
3 cups Edita's Fountain of Youth Salad
2 tablespoons nonfat salad dressing
Black coffee or tea and 8 ounces water

Bedtime Snack

1 slice raisin bread
1 cup Edita's Fountain of Youth Fruit Salad

DAY 31

Breakfast

1 cup Total® cereal
½ cup skim milk
1 orange

Black coffee or tea and 8 ounces water

Morning Snack

½ cantaloupe

Lunch

2 slices low-calorie whole wheat bread
1 tomato
1 ounce skim milk mozzarella cheese
3 cups Edita's Fountain of Youth Salad
2 tablespoons nonfat salad dressing
Black coffee or tea and 8 ounces water

Afternoon Snack

1 cup nonfat fruit-flavored yogurt
½ cantaloupe

Dinner

4 ounces skinless chicken breast, baked, broiled, or grilled
4 cups Edita's Fountain of Youth Veggies, steamed
3 cups Edita's Fountain of Youth Salad
2 tablespoons nonfat salad dressing
Black coffee or tea and 8 ounces water

Bedtime Snack

2 slices low-calorie whole wheat bread
1 teaspoon all-fruit preserves
1 cup skim milk

DAY 32

Breakfast
1 bagel
1 teaspoon all-fruit preserves
Black coffee or tea and 8 ounces
    water

Morning Snack
1 cup Edita's Fountain of Youth
    Fruit Salad

Lunch
4 ounces tuna (packed in water)
3 cups Edita's Fountain of Youth
    Salad
2 tablespoons nonfat salad
    dressing
Black coffee or tea and 8 ounces
    water

Afternoon Snack
1 cup Edita's Fountain of Youth
    Fruit Salad

Dinner
1 baked potato
4 cups Edita's Fountain of Youth
    Veggies, steamed
4 cups Edita's Fountain of Youth
    Salad
1 cup nonfat plain yogurt
½ cup salsa
Black coffee or tea and 8 ounces
    water

Bedtime Snack
2 slices low-calorie whole wheat
    bread

1 teaspoon all-fruit preserves
1 cup skim milk

DAY 33

Breakfast
1 English muffin
2 teaspoons all-fruit preserves
1 orange
Black coffee or tea and 8 ounces
    water

Morning Snack
1 cup carrots
1 cup celery
½ cup plain nonfat yogurt
¼ cup salsa

Lunch
2 slices low-calorie whole wheat
    bread
1 hard-boiled egg
3 cups Edita's Fountain of Youth
    Salad
2 tablespoons nonfat salad
    dressing
Black coffee or tea and 8 ounces
    water

Afternoon Snack
1 cup Edita's Fountain of Youth
    Fruit Salad
1 fig cookie

Dinner
4 ounces white turkey meat
1 cup brussels sprouts
1 sweet potato

3 cups Edita's Fountain of Youth
Salad
2 tablespoons nonfat salad
dressing
Black coffee or tea and 8 ounces
water

Bedtime Snack
2 rice cakes
1 teaspoon honey
1 cup skim milk

DAY 34

Breakfast
1 cup oatmeal
1 tablespoon brown sugar
1 grapefruit
Black coffee or tea and 8 ounces
water

Morning Snack
½ cantaloupe

Lunch
1 rice cake
1 cup tomato soup made with
water
3 cups Edita's Fountain of Youth
Salad
2 tablespoons nonfat salad
dressing
Black coffee or tea and 8 ounces
water

Afternoon Snack
1 cup air-popped popcorn

1 teaspoon grated Parmesan
cheese

Dinner
4 ounces flounder, broiled, baked,
or grilled
1 baked potato
3 cups Edita's Fountain of Youth
Salad
2 tablespoons nonfat salad
dressing
Black coffee or tea and 8 ounces
water

Bedtime Snack
1 cup raisin bran
½ cup skim milk

DAY 35

Breakfast
2 slices low-calorie whole wheat
bread
2 teaspoons all-fruit preserves
Black coffee or tea and 8 ounces
water

Morning Snack
1 cup vegetable juice
2 rice cakes

Lunch
1 bagel
1 teaspoon cream cheese
2 ounces smoked salmon
1 tomato
½ Bermuda onion, sliced

Black coffee or tea and 8 ounces
water

Afternoon Snack
1 cup nonfat fruit yogurt

Dinner
1 baked potato
4 cups Edita's Fountain of Youth
Veggies, steamed
½ cup salsa
3 cups Edita's Fountain of Youth
Salad
2 tablespoons nonfat salad
dressing
Black coffee or tea and 8 ounces
water

Bedtime Snack
1 cup Edita's Fountain of Youth
Fruit Salad

DAY 36

Breakfast
1 cup strawberries
1 cup nonfat fruit yogurt
½ cup raisin bran
Black coffee or tea and 8 ounces
water

Morning Snack
2 rice cakes
2 teaspoons all-fruit preserves

Lunch
2 slices low-calorie whole wheat
bread

1 ounce low-fat Cheddar cheese
3 cups Edita's Fountain of Youth
Salad
2 tablespoons nonfat salad
dressing
Black coffee or tea and 8 ounces
water

Afternoon Snack
½ cantaloupe

Dinner
1 cup cooked spaghetti
½ cup spaghetti sauce
1 teaspoon grated Parmesan
cheese
3 cups Edita's Fountain of Youth
Salad
2 tablespoons nonfat salad
dressing
Black coffee or tea and 8 ounces
water

Bedtime Snack
1 slice low-calorie whole wheat
bread
1 teaspoon all-fruit preserves
1 cup skim milk

DAY 37

Breakfast
3 blueberry pancakes
2 tablespoons maple syrup
Black coffee or tea and 8 ounces
water

Morning Snack
1 apple
½ cup carrots
½ cup celery

Lunch
1 pita bread
1 tomato
¼ Bermuda onion, sliced
3 cups Edita's Fountain of Youth
    Salad
2 tablespoons nonfat salad
    dressing
Black coffee or tea and 8 ounces
    water

Afternoon Snack
1 cup air-popped popcorn
1 teaspoon grated Parmesan
    cheese

Dinner
4 cups Edita's Fountain of Youth
    Veggies, steamed
1 baked potato
3 cups Edita's Fountain of Youth
    Salad
2 tablespoons nonfat salad
    dressing
Black coffee or tea and 8 ounces
    water

Bedtime Snack
½ cantaloupe

DAY 38

Breakfast
1 bagel
1 teaspoon all-fruit preserves

Black coffee or tea and 8 ounces
    water

Morning Snack
1 cup nonfat fruit yogurt

Lunch
4 ounces tuna (packed in water)
2 slices low-calorie whole wheat
    bread
3 cups Edita's Fountain of Youth
    Salad
2 tablespoons nonfat salad
    dressing
Black coffee or tea and 8 ounces
    water

Afternoon Snack
1 rice cake
1 ounce low-fat Swiss cheese
1 sweet red pepper

Dinner
4 ounces skinless chicken breast,
    baked, broiled, or grilled
1 sweet potato, baked
4 cups Edita's Fountain of Youth
    Veggies, steamed
Black coffee or tea and 8 ounces
    water

Bedtime Snack
1 cup raisin bran
½ cup skim milk

DAY 39

Breakfast
1 English muffin
1 cup nonfat fruit yogurt

Black coffee or tea and 8 ounces
water

Morning Snack
1 cup Edita's Fountain of Youth
Fruit Salad

Lunch
1 pita bread
1 tomato
½ cucumber
¼ Bermuda onion
¼ cup salsa
Black coffee or tea and 8 ounces
water

Afternoon Snack
1 cup air-popped popcorn
1 teaspoon grated Parmesan
cheese

Dinner
1 baked potato
1 ounce low-fat Cheddar cheese
3 cups Edita's Fountain of Youth
Salad
4 cups Edita's Fountain of Youth
Veggies, steamed
Black coffee or tea and 8 ounces
water

Bedtime Snack
1 cup Edita's Fountain of Youth
Fruit Salad

Day 40

Breakfast
1 cup oatmeal
1 tablespoon brown sugar

1 orange
Black coffee or tea and 8 ounces
water

Morning Snack
1 cup nonfat fruit yogurt

Lunch
1 cup chicken noodle soup
3 cups Edita's Fountain of Youth
Salad
2 tablespoons nonfat salad
dressing
Black coffee or tea and 8 ounces
water

Afternoon Snack
1 slice low-calorie whole wheat
bread
1 tomato

Dinner
4 ounces salmon
1 baked potato
4 cups Edita's Fountain of Youth
Veggies, steamed
Black coffee or tea and 8 ounces
water

Bedtime Snack
1 cup Edita's Fountain of Youth
Fruit Salad

Day 41

Breakfast
1 cup Total® cereal
½ cup skim milk
1 cup Edita's Fountain of Youth
Fruit Salad

Black coffee or tea and 8 ounces
water

Morning Snack
1 cup nonfat fruit yogurt

Lunch
4 ounces skinless turkey breast
2 slices low-calorie whole wheat
bread
1 tomato
Black coffee or tea and 8 ounces
water

Afternoon Snack
1 apple
1 cup carrots
1 cup celery

Dinner
1 cup spaghetti
½ cup spaghetti sauce
1 teaspoon grated Parmesan
cheese
3 cups Edita's Fountain of Youth
Salad
2 tablespoons nonfat salad
dressing
Black coffee or tea and 8 ounces
water

Bedtime Snack
1 slice low-calorie whole wheat
bread
1 teaspoon all-fruit preserves

DAY 42

Breakfast
1 cup nonfat fruit yogurt
½ cup raisin bran
1 cup Edita's Fountain of Youth
Salad
Black coffee or tea and 8 ounces
water

Morning Snack
1 cup carrots
1 cup celery
1 red pepper

Lunch
1 cup vegetable soup
2 rice cakes
1 teaspoon cream cheese
Black coffee or tea and 8 ounces
water

Afternoon Snack
1 cup Edita's Fountain of Youth
Fruit Salad

Dinner
4 ounces skinless turkey breast,
baked, broiled, or grilled
4 cups Edita's Fountain of Youth
Veggies, steamed
3 cups Edita's Fountain of Youth
Salad
2 tablespoons nonfat salad
dressing
Black coffee or tea and 8 ounces
water

Bedtime Snack

1 slice low-calorie whole wheat
  bread
1 teaspoon honey

DAY 43

Breakfast

2 slices French toast
2 tablespoons maple syrup
Black coffee or tea and 8 ounces
  water

Morning Snack

1 cup Edita's Fountain of Youth
  Fruit Salad

Lunch

4 ounces tuna (packed in water)
3 cups Edita's Fountain of Youth
  Salad
2 tablespoons nonfat salad
  dressing
Black coffee or tea and 8 ounces
  water

Afternoon Snack

1 cup air-popped popcorn
¼ cup raisins

Dinner

4 ounces flounder, baked, broiled,
  or grilled
4 cups Edita's Fountain of Youth
  Veggies, steamed
3 cups Edita's Fountain of Youth
  Salad

2 tablespoons nonfat salad
  dressing
Black coffee or tea and 8 ounces
  water

Bedtime Snack

2 slices low-calorie whole wheat
  bread
2 teaspoons all-fruit preserves

DAY 44

Breakfast

1 bagel
1 egg
1 sliced tomato
Black coffee or tea and 8 ounces
  water

Morning Snack

1 cup vegetable juice
½ cup carrots
½ cup celery

Lunch

1 hamburger patty, grilled or
  broiled
3 cups Edita's Fountain of Youth
  Salad
2 tablespoons nonfat salad
  dressing
Black coffee or tea and 8 ounces
  water

Afternoon Snack

1 cup Edita's Fountain of Youth
  Fruit Salad

Dinner
4 cups Edita's Fountain of Youth
   Veggies, steamed
1 baked potato
¼ cup salsa
Black coffee or tea and 8 ounces
   water

Bedtime Snack
1 cup skim milk
1 slice raisin bread

Day 45

Breakfast
1 cup Total® cereal
½ cup skim milk
1 grapefruit
Black coffee or tea and 8 ounces
   water

Morning Snack
2 rice cakes
2 teaspoons all-fruit preserves

Lunch
1 pita bread
1 tomato
¼ cup lettuce
1 ounce low-fat Cheddar cheese
Black coffee or tea and 8 ounces
   water

Afternoon Snack
½ cup nonfat fruit yogurt
½ cup raisin bran

Dinner
4 ounces canned salmon
4 cups Edita's Fountain of Youth
   Veggies, steamed
3 cups Edita's Fountain of Youth
   Salad
1 baked potato
2 tablespoons nonfat salad
   dressing
Black coffee or tea and 8 ounces
   water

Bedtime Snack
1 cup Edita's Fountain of Youth
   Fruit Salad
1 fig cookie

Day 46

Breakfast
2 slices low-calorie whole wheat
   bread
1 tomato
1 ounce low-fat Cheddar cheese
Black coffee or tea and 8 ounces
   water

Morning Snack
1 cup Edita's Fountain of Youth
   Fruit Salad

Lunch
4 ounces tuna (packed in water)
1 tomato
½ cup plain nonfat yogurt
¼ cup salsa ·
Black coffee or tea and 8 ounces
   water

Afternoon Snack

3 cups Edita's Fountain of Youth
Salad
1 slice low-calorie whole wheat
bread
2 tablespoons nonfat salad
dressing

Dinner

1 sweet potato, baked
4 ounces chicken breast, broiled,
baked, or grilled
3 cups Edita's Fountain of Youth
Salad
2 tablespoons nonfat salad
dressing
Black coffee or tea and 8 ounces
water

Bedtime Snack

1 cup Total® cereal
½ cup skim milk

DAY 47

Breakfast

1 cup oatmeal
2 teaspoons maple syrup
1 orange
Black coffee or tea and 8 ounces
water

Morning Snack

1 cup nonfat fruit yogurt
½ cup raisin bran

Lunch

2 slices low-calorie whole wheat
bread

2 ounces sliced turkey breast
3 cups Edita's Fountain of Youth
Salad
2 tablespoons nonfat salad
dressing
Black coffee or tea and 8 ounces
water

Afternoon Snack

2 rice cakes
2 teaspoons all-fruit preserves

Dinner

1 baked potato
1 teaspoon grated Parmesan
cheese
4 cups Edita's Fountain of Youth
Veggies, steamed
½ cup nonfat plain yogurt
¼ cup salsa
Black coffee or tea and 8 ounces
water

Bedtime Snack

1 cup Edita's Fountain of Youth
Fruit Salad
1 slice raisin bread

DAY 48

Breakfast

1 English muffin
2 teaspoons all-fruit preserves
1 cup Edita's Fountain of Youth
Fruit Salad
Black coffee or tea and 8 ounces
water

Morning Snack
½ cup carrots
½ cup red and green peppers
1 rice cake

Lunch
1 egg
2 slices low-calorie whole wheat
  bread
1 tomato
½ Bermuda onion
2 tablespoons nonfat salad
  dressing
Black coffee or tea and 8 ounces
  water

Afternoon Snack
1 cup air-popped popcorn
1 teaspoon grated Parmesan
  cheese

Dinner
1 cup spaghetti
½ cup tomato sauce
3 cups Edita's Fountain of Youth
  Salad
2 tablespoons nonfat salad
  dressing
Black coffee or tea and 8 ounces
  water

Bedtime Snack
1 cup Edita's Fountain of Youth
  Fruit Salad

DAY 49

Breakfast
1 bagel
2 teaspoons cream cheese

2 teaspoons all-fruit preserves
Black coffee or tea and 8 ounces
  water

Morning Snack
1 cup Edita's Fountain of Youth
  Fruit Salad
1 cup nonfat fruit yogurt

Lunch
3 cups Edita's Fountain of Youth
  Salad
4 ounces canned salmon
2 tablespoons nonfat salad
  dressing
Black coffee or tea and 8 ounces
  water

Afternoon Snack
1 cup Edita's Fountain of Youth
  Fruit Salad

Dinner
1 baked potato
1 teaspoon grated Parmesan
  cheese
3 cups Edita's Fountain of Youth
  Salad
2 tablespoons nonfat salad
  dressing
4 cups Edita's Fountain of Youth
  Veggies, steamed
½ cup nonfat plain yogurt
¼ cup salsa
Black coffee or tea and 8 ounces
  water

Bedtime Snack
2 slices low-calorie whole wheat
  bread
2 tablespoons all-fruit preserves

DAY 50

Breakfast
1 cup Total® cereal
½ cup skim milk
1 grapefruit
Black coffee or tea and 8 ounces
    water

Morning Snack
2 rice cakes
2 teaspoons all-fruit preserves

Lunch
2 slices low-calorie whole wheat
    bread
1 tomato
½ Bermuda onion
3 cups Edita's Fountain of Youth
    Salad
2 tablespoons nonfat salad
    dressing
Black coffee or tea and 8 ounces
    water

Afternoon Snack
1 apple
1 ounce low-fat Cheddar cheese

Dinner
3 cups Edita's Fountain of Youth
    Salad
2 tablespoons nonfat salad
    dressing
4 cups Edita's Fountain of Youth
    Veggies, steamed
½ cup nonfat plain yogurt
¼ cup salsa
1 baked potato

Black coffee or tea and 8 ounces
    water

Bedtime Snack
1 cup Edita's Fountain of Youth
    Fruit Salad
1 slice raisin bread

DAY 51

Breakfast
3 buttermilk pancakes
2 tablespoons maple syrup
Black coffee or tea and 8 ounces
    water

Morning Snack
½ cup carrots
½ cup celery

Lunch
1 baked potato
½ cup nonfat plain yogurt
¼ cup salsa
Black coffee or tea and 8 ounces
    water

Afternoon Snack
1 cup air-popped popcorn
1 teaspoon grated Parmesan
    cheese

Dinner
1 ground beef patty, broiled or
    grilled
2 cups Edita's Fountain of Youth
    Salad
2 tablespoons nonfat salad
    dressing

4 cups Edita's Fountain of Youth
    Veggies, steamed
Black coffee or tea and 8 ounces
    water

Bedtime Snack
1 apple
1 fig cookie

DAY 52

Breakfast
1 cup nonfat fruit yogurt
½ cup Total® cereal
Black coffee or tea and 8 ounces
    water

Morning Snack
1 cup Edita's Fountain of Youth
    Fruit Salad

Lunch
2 slices low-calorie whole wheat
    bread
1 ounce low-fat Cheddar cheese
1 tomato
½ Bermuda onion
2 tablespoons nonfat salad
    dressing
Black coffee or tea and 8 ounces
    water

Afternoon Snack
½ cantaloupe

Dinner
4 ounces skinless chicken breast,
    baked, broiled, or grilled
1 cup stuffing
3 cups Edita's Fountain of Youth
    Salad
2 tablespoons nonfat salad
    dressing
Black coffee or tea and 8 ounces
    water

Bedtime Snack
1 bagel
2 teaspoons all-fruit preserves

DAY 53

Breakfast
½ cantaloupe
2 slices low-calorie whole wheat
    bread
2 teaspoons all-fruit preserves
Black coffee or tea and 8 ounces
    water

Morning Snack
1 grapefruit
1 cup nonfat fruit yogurt

Lunch
1 egg
3 cups Edita's Fountain of Youth
    Salad
2 tablespoons nonfat salad
    dressing
Black coffee or tea and 8 ounces
    water

Afternoon Snack
2 rice cakes
2 teaspoons all-fruit preserves

Dinner
4 cups Edita's Fountain of Youth Veggies, steamed
3 cups Edita's Fountain of Youth Salad
2 tablespoons nonfat salad dressing
1 baked potato
Black coffee or tea and 8 ounces water

Bedtime Snack
1 cup Edita's Fountain of Youth Fruit Salad

DAY 54

Breakfast
1 cup oatmeal
1 tablespoon brown sugar
1 grapefruit
Black coffee or tea and 8 ounces water

Morning Snack
½ cantaloupe

Lunch
1 rice cake
1 cup tomato soup made with water
3 cups Edita's Fountain of Youth Salad

2 tablespoons nonfat salad dressing
Black coffee or tea and 8 ounces water

Afternoon Snack
1 cup air-popped popcorn
1 teaspoon grated Parmesan cheese

Dinner
4 ounces flounder, broiled, baked, or grilled
1 baked potato
3 cups Edita's Fountain of Youth Salad
2 tablespoons nonfat salad dressing
Black coffee or tea and 8 ounces water

Bedtime Snack
1 cup Total® cereal
½ cup skim milk

DAY 55

Breakfast
2 slices French toast
2 tablespoons maple syrup
Black coffee or tea and 8 ounces water

Morning Snack
1 cup nonfat fruit yogurt

Lunch
1 cup vegetable soup
3 cups Edita's Fountain of Youth
   Salad
2 tablespoons nonfat salad
   dressing
Black coffee or tea and 8 ounces
   water

Afternoon Snack
1 slice low-calorie whole wheat
   bread
1 tomato

Dinner
4 ounces salmon, broiled, baked,
   or poached
1 baked potato
4 cups Edita's Fountain of Youth
   Veggies, steamed
Black coffee or tea and 8 ounces
   water

Bedtime Snack
1 cup Edita's Fountain of Youth
   Fruit Salad

DAY 56

Breakfast
1 English muffin
1 cup nonfat fruit yogurt
Black coffee or tea and 8 ounces
   water

Morning Snack
1 cup Edita's Fountain of Youth
   Fruit Salad

Lunch
1 pita bread
1 tomato
½ cucumber
¼ Bermuda onion
¼ cup salsa
Black coffee or tea and 8 ounces
   water

Afternoon Snack
1 apple
1 cup carrots
1 cup celery

Dinner
1 cup spaghetti
½ cup spaghetti sauce
1 teaspoon grated Parmesan
   cheese
3 cups Edita's Fountain of Youth
   Salad
2 tablespoons nonfat salad
   dressing
Black coffee or tea and 8 ounces
   water

Bedtime Snack
1 slice low-calorie whole wheat
   bread
1 teaspoon all-fruit preserves

DAY 57

Breakfast
1 slice low-calorie whole wheat
  bread
1 teaspoon all-fruit preserves
1 cup Edita's Fountain of Youth
  Fruit Salad
Black coffee or tea and 8 ounces
  water

Morning Snack
1 cup vegetable juice
2 rice cakes

Lunch
1 bagel
1 tablespoon cream cheese
2 ounces smoked salmon
1 tomato
½ Bermuda onion, sliced
Black coffee or tea and 8 ounces
  water

Afternoon Snack
1 cup nonfat fruit yogurt

Dinner
4 cups Edita's Fountain of Youth
  Veggies, steamed
½ cup plain nonfat yogurt
¼ cup salsa
3 cups Edita's Fountain of Youth
  Salad
2 tablespoons nonfat salad
  dressing
Black coffee or tea and 8 ounces
  water

Bedtime Snack
1 cup Edita's Fountain of Youth
  Fruit Salad
1 fig cookie

DAY 58

Breakfast
1 cup strawberries
1 cup nonfat fruit yogurt
½ cup raisin bran
Black coffee or tea and 8 ounces
  water

Morning Snack
2 rice cakes
2 teaspoons all-fruit preserves

Lunch
2 slices low-calorie whole wheat
  bread
1 ounce low-fat Cheddar cheese
3 cups Edita's Fountain of Youth
  Salad
2 tablespoons nonfat salad
  dressing
Black coffee or tea and 8 ounces
  water

Afternoon Snack
½ cantaloupe

Dinner
4 ounces flounder, baked, broiled,
  or grilled
1 sweet potato, baked
3 cups Edita's Fountain of Youth
  Salad

2 tablespoons nonfat salad
   dressing
Black coffee or tea and 8 ounces
   water

Bedtime Snack
1 slice low-calorie whole wheat
   bread
1 teaspoon all-fruit preserves
1 cup skim milk

DAY 59

Breakfast
1 bagel
1 teaspoon all-fruit preserves
Black coffee or tea and 8 ounces
   water

Morning Snack
½ cantaloupe

Lunch
4 ounces tuna (packed in water)
3 cups Edita's Fountain of Youth
   Salad
2 tablespoons nonfat salad
   dressing
Black coffee or tea and 8 ounces
   water

Afternoon Snack
1 cup Edita's Fountain of Youth
   Fruit Salad

Dinner
1 baked potato
4 cups Edita's Fountain of Youth
   Veggies, steamed
1 cup plain yogurt
½ cup salsa
3 cups Edita's Fountain of Youth
   Salad
2 tablespoons nonfat salad
   dressing
Black coffee or tea and 8 ounces
   water

Bedtime Snack
1 slice low-calorie whole wheat
   bread
1 teaspoon honey
1 cup skim milk

DAY 60

Breakfast
3 blueberry pancakes
2 tablespoons maple syrup
Black coffee or tea and 8 ounces
   water

Morning Snack
1 apple
2 rice cakes

Lunch
1 pita bread
1 tomato
¼ Bermuda onion
3 cups Edita's Fountain of Youth
   Salad

2 tablespoons nonfat salad
dressing
Black coffee or tea and 8 ounces
water

Afternoon Snack
1 cup air-popped popcorn
1 teaspoon grated Parmesan
cheese

Dinner
4 ounces skinless chicken breast,
broiled, baked, or grilled
1 baked potato
3 cups Edita's Fountain of Youth
Salad
2 tablespoons nonfat salad
dressing
Black coffee or tea and 8 ounces
water

Bedtime Snack
1 slice raisin bread
1 cup Edita's Fountain of Youth
Fruit Salad

Day 61

Breakfast
1 cup Total® cereal
½ cup skim milk
1 orange
Black coffee or tea and 8 ounces
water

Morning Snack
½ cantaloupe

Lunch
2 slices low-calorie whole wheat
bread
1 tomato
1 ounce skim milk mozzarella
cheese
3 cups Edita's Fountain of Youth
Salad
2 tablespoons nonfat salad
dressing
Black coffee or tea and 8 ounces
water

Afternoon Snack
1 cup nonfat fruit-flavored yogurt
½ cantaloupe

Dinner
4 ounces skinless chicken breast,
broiled, baked, or grilled
4 cups Edita's Fountain of Youth
Veggies, steamed
3 cups Edita's Fountain of Youth
Salad
2 tablespoons nonfat salad
dressing
Black coffee or tea and 8 ounces
water

Bedtime Snack
2 slices low-calorie whole wheat
bread
1 teaspoon all-fruit preserves
1 cup skim milk

DAY 62

Breakfast
1 bagel
1 teaspoon all-fruit preserves
Black coffee or tea and 8 ounces
    water

Morning Snack
1 cup Edita's Fountain of Youth
    Fruit Salad

Lunch
4 ounces tuna (packed in water)
3 cups Edita's Fountain of Youth
    Salad
2 tablespoons nonfat salad
    dressing
Black coffee or tea and 8 ounces
    water

Afternoon Snack
1 cup Edita's Fountain of Youth
    Fruit Salad

Dinner
1 baked potato
4 cups Edita's Fountain of Youth
    Veggies, steamed
4 cups Edita's Fountain of Youth
    Salad
1 cup nonfat plain yogurt
½ cup salsa
Black coffee or tea and 8 ounces
    water

Bedtime Snack
2 slices low-calorie whole wheat
    bread

1 teaspoon all-fruit preserves
1 cup skim milk

DAY 63

Breakfast
1 English muffin
2 teaspoons all-fruit preserves
1 orange
Black coffee or tea and 8 ounces
    water

Morning Snack
1 cup carrots
1 cup celery
½ cup plain nonfat yogurt
¼ cup salsa

Lunch
2 slices low-calorie whole wheat
    bread
1 egg
3 cups Edita's Fountain of Youth
    Salad
Black coffee or tea and 8 ounces
    water

Afternoon Snack
1 cup Edita's Fountain of Youth
    Fruit Salad
1 fig cookie

Dinner
4 ounces white meat turkey,
    broiled, baked, or grilled
1 cup brussels sprouts
1 sweet potato

3 cups Edita's Fountain of Youth
    Salad
2 tablespoons nonfat salad
    dressing
Black coffee or tea and 8 ounces
    water

Bedtime Snack
2 rice cakes
1 teaspoon honey
1 cup skim milk

DAY 64

Breakfast
1 cup oatmeal
1 tablespoon brown sugar
1 grapefruit
Black coffee or tea and 8 ounces
    water

Morning Snack
½ cantaloupe

Lunch
1 rice cake
1 cup tomato soup made with
    water
3 cups Edita's Fountain of Youth
    Salad
2 tablespoons nonfat salad
    dressing
Black coffee or tea and 8 ounces
    water

Afternoon Snack
1 cup air-popped popcorn

1 teaspoon grated Parmesan
    cheese

Dinner
4 ounces flounder, broiled, baked,
    or grilled
1 baked potato
3 cups Edita's Fountain of Youth
    Salad
2 tablespoons nonfat salad
    dressing
Black coffee or tea and 8 ounces
    water

Bedtime Snack
1 cup raisin bran
½ cup skim milk

DAY 65

Breakfast
2 slices low-calorie whole wheat
    bread
2 teaspoons all-fruit preserves
Black coffee or tea and 8 ounces
    water

Morning Snack
1 cup vegetable juice
2 rice cakes

Lunch
½ bagel
1 teaspoon cream cheese
2 ounces smoked salmon
1 tomato
½ Bermuda onion, sliced

Black coffee or tea and 8 ounces
water

Afternoon Snack
1 cup nonfat fruit yogurt

Dinner
1 baked potato
4 cups Edita's Fountain of Youth
Veggies, steamed
½ cup salsa
3 cups Edita's Fountain of Youth
Salad
2 tablespoons nonfat salad
dressing
Black coffee or tea and 8 ounces
water

Bedtime Snack
1 cup Edita's Fountain of Youth
Fruit Salad

DAY 66

Breakfast
1 cup strawberries
1 cup nonfat fruit yogurt
½ cup raisin bran
Black coffee or tea and 8 ounces
water

Morning Snack
2 rice cakes
2 teaspoons all-fruit preserves

Lunch
2 slices low-calorie whole wheat
bread

1 ounce low-fat Cheddar cheese
3 cups Edita's Fountain of Youth
Salad
2 tablespoons nonfat salad
dressing
Black coffee or tea and 8 ounces
water

Afternoon Snack
½ cantaloupe

Dinner
1 cup cooked spaghetti
½ cup spaghetti sauce
1 teaspoon grated Parmesan
cheese
3 cups Edita's Fountain of Youth
Salad
2 tablespoons nonfat salad
dressing
Black coffee or tea and 8 ounces
water

Bedtime Snack
1 slice low-calorie whole wheat
bread
1 teaspoon all-fruit preserves
1 cup skim milk

DAY 67

Breakfast
3 blueberry pancakes
2 tablespoons maple syrup
Black coffee or tea and 8 ounces
water

Morning Snack
1 apple
½ cup carrots
½ cup celery

Lunch
1 pita bread
1 tomato
½ Bermuda onion, sliced
3 cups Edita's Fountain of Youth
Salad
2 tablespoons nonfat salad
dressing
Black coffee or tea and 8 ounces
water

Afternoon Snack
1 cup air-popped popcorn
1 teaspoon grated Parmesan
cheese

Dinner
4 cups Edita's Fountain of Youth
Veggies, steamed
1 baked potato
3 cups Edita's Fountain of Youth
Salad
2 tablespoons nonfat salad
dressing
Black coffee or tea and 8 ounces
water

Bedtime Snack
½ cantaloupe

DAY 68

Breakfast
1 bagel
1 teaspoon all-fruit preserves
Black coffee or tea and 8 ounces
water

Morning Snack
1 cup nonfat fruit yogurt

Lunch
4 ounces tuna (packed in water)
2 slices low-calorie whole wheat
bread
3 cups Edita's Fountain of Youth
Salad
2 tablespoons nonfat salad
dressing
Black coffee or tea and 8 ounces
water

Afternoon Snack
1 rice cake
1 ounce low-fat Swiss cheese
1 sweet red pepper

Dinner
4 ounces skinless chicken breast,
baked or broiled
1 sweet potato, baked
4 cups Edita's Fountain of Youth
Veggies, steamed
Black coffee or tea and 8 ounces
water

Bedtime Snack

1 cup raisin bran

½ cup skim milk

DAY 69

Breakfast

1 English muffin

1 cup nonfat fruit yogurt

Black coffee or tea and 8 ounces
water

Morning Snack

1 cup Edita's Fountain of Youth
Fruit Salad

Lunch

1 pita bread

1 tomato

½ cucumber

¼ Bermuda onion

¼ cup salsa

Black coffee or tea and 8 ounces
water

Afternoon Snack

1 cup air-popped popcorn

1 teaspoon grated Parmesan
cheese

Dinner

1 baked potato

1 ounce low-fat Cheddar cheese

3 cups Edita's Fountain of Youth
Salad

4 cups Edita's Fountain of Youth
Veggies, steamed

Black coffee or tea and 8 ounces
water

Bedtime Snack

1 cup Edita's Fountain of Youth
Fruit Salad

DAY 70

Breakfast

1 cup oatmeal

1 tablespoon brown sugar

1 orange

Black coffee or tea and 8 ounces
water

Morning Snack

1 cup nonfat fruit yogurt

Lunch

1 cup chicken noodle soup

3 cups Edita's Fountain of Youth
Salad

2 tablespoons nonfat salad
dressing

Black coffee or tea and 8 ounces
water

Afternoon Snack

1 slice low-calorie whole wheat
bread

1 tomato

Dinner
4 ounces salmon, baked, broiled,
    grilled, or poached
1 baked potato
4 cups Edita's Fountain of Youth
    Veggies, steamed
Black coffee or tea and 8 ounces
    water

Bedtime Snack
1 cup Edita's Fountain of Youth
    Fruit Salad

Day 71

Breakfast
1 cup Total® cereal
½ cup skim milk
1 cup Edita's Fountain of Youth
    Fruit Salad
Black coffee or tea and 8 ounces
    water

Morning Snack
1 cup nonfat fruit yogurt

Lunch
4 ounces skinless turkey breast,
    baked, broiled, or grilled
2 slices low-calorie whole wheat
    bread
1 tomato
Black coffee or tea and 8 ounces
    water

Afternoon Snack
1 apple
1 cup carrots
1 cup celery

Dinner
1 cup spaghetti
½ cup spaghetti sauce
1 teaspoon grated Parmesan
    cheese
3 cups Edita's Fountain of Youth
    Salad
2 tablespoons nonfat salad
    dressing
Black coffee or tea and 8 ounces
    water

Bedtime Snack
1 slice low-calorie whole wheat
    bread
1 teaspoon all-fruit preserves

Day 72

Breakfast
1 cup nonfat fruit yogurt
½ cup raisin bran
1 cup Edita's Fountain of Youth
    Fruit Salad
Black coffee or tea and 8 ounces
    water

Morning Snack
1 cup carrots
1 cup celery
1 red pepper

Lunch

1 cup vegetable soup
2 rice cakes
1 teaspoon cream cheese
Black coffee or tea and 8 ounces
    water

Afternoon Snack

1 cup Edita's Fountain of Youth
    Fruit Salad

Dinner

4 ounces skinless turkey breast,
    baked, broiled, or grilled
4 cups Edita's Fountain of Youth
    Veggies, steamed
3 cups Edita's Fountain of Youth
    Salad
2 tablespoons nonfat salad
    dressing
Black coffee or tea and 8 ounces
    water

Bedtime Snack

1 slice low-calorie whole wheat
    bread
1 teaspoon honey

DAY 73

Breakfast

2 slices French toast
2 tablespoons maple syrup
Black coffee or tea and 8 ounces
    water

Morning Snack

1 cup Edita's Fountain of Youth
    Fruit Salad

Lunch

4 ounces tuna (packed in water)
3 cups Edita's Fountain of Youth
    Salad
2 tablespoons nonfat salad
    dressing
Black coffee or tea and 8 ounces
    water

Afternoon Snack

1 cup air-popped popcorn
¼ cup raisins

Dinner

4 ounces flounder, baked, broiled,
    or grilled
4 cups Edita's Fountain of Youth
    Veggies, steamed
3 cups Edita's Fountain of Youth
    Salad
2 tablespoons nonfat salad
    dressing
Black coffee or tea and 8 ounces
    water

Bedtime Snack

2 slices low-calorie whole wheat
    bread
2 teaspoons all-fruit preserves

DAY 74

Breakfast

1 bagel
1 egg
1 sliced tomato
Black coffee or tea and 8 ounces
    water

Morning Snack
1 cup vegetable juice
½ cup carrots
½ cup celery

Lunch
1 hamburger patty, grilled or
  broiled
3 cups Edita's Fountain of Youth
  Salad
2 tablespoons nonfat salad
  dressing
Black coffee or tea and 8 ounces
  water

Afternoon Snack
1 cup Edita's Fountain of Youth
  Fruit Salad

Dinner
4 cups Edita's Fountain of Youth
  Veggies, steamed
1 baked potato
¼ cup salsa

Bedtime Snack
1 cup skim milk
1 slice raisin bread

DAY 75

Breakfast
1 cup Total® cereal
½ cup skim milk
1 grapefruit
Black coffee or tea and 8 ounces
  water

Morning Snack
2 rice cakes
2 teaspoons all-fruit preserves

Lunch
1 pita bread
1 tomato
¼ cup lettuce
1 ounce low-fat Cheddar cheese
Black coffee or tea and 8 ounces
  water

Afternoon Snack
½ cup nonfat fruit yogurt
½ cup raisin bran

Dinner
4 ounces canned salmon
4 cups Edita's Fountain of Youth
  Veggies, steamed
3 cups Edita's Fountain of Youth
  Salad
1 baked potato
2 tablespoons nonfat salad
  dressing
Black coffee or tea and 8 ounces
  water

Bedtime Snack
1 cup Edita's Fountain of Youth
  Fruit Salad
1 fig cookie

DAY 76

Breakfast
2 slices low-calorie whole wheat
  bread
1 tomato

1 ounce low-fat Cheddar cheese
Black coffee or tea and 8 ounces
    water

Morning Snack
1 cup Edita's Fountain of Youth
    Fruit Salad

Lunch
4 ounces tuna (packed in water)
1 tomato
½ cup plain nonfat yogurt
¼ cup salsa
Black coffee or tea and 8 ounces
    water

Afternoon Snack
3 cups Edita's Fountain of Youth
    Salad
1 slice low-calorie whole wheat
    bread
2 tablespoons nonfat salad
    dressing

Dinner
1 sweet potato, baked
4 ounces chicken breast, broiled,
    baked, or grilled
3 cups Edita's Fountain of Youth
    Salad
2 tablespoons nonfat salad
    dressing
Black coffee or tea and 8 ounces
    water

Bedtime Snack
1 cup Total® cereal
½ cup skim milk

DAY 77

Breakfast
1 cup oatmeal
2 teaspoons maple syrup
1 orange
Black coffee or tea and 8 ounces
    water

Morning Snack
1 cup nonfat fruit yogurt
½ cup raisin bran

Lunch
2 slices low-calorie whole wheat
    bread
2 ounces sliced turkey breast
3 cups Edita's Fountain of Youth
    Salad
2 tablespoons nonfat salad
    dressing
Black coffee or tea and 8 ounces
    water

Afternoon Snack
2 rice cakes
2 teaspoons all-fruit preserves

Dinner
1 baked potato
1 teaspoon grated Parmesan
    cheese
4 cups Edita's Fountain of Youth
    Veggies, steamed
½ cup nonfat plain yogurt
¼ cup salsa

Black coffee or tea and 8 ounces
water

Bedtime Snack
1 cup Edita's Fountain of Youth
Fruit Salad
1 slice raisin bread

DAY 78

Breakfast
1 English muffin
2 teaspoons all-fruit preserves
1 cup Edita's Fountain of Youth
Fruit Salad
Black coffee or tea and 8 ounces
water

Morning Snack
½ cup carrots
½ cup red and green peppers
1 rice cake

Lunch
1 egg
2 slices low-calorie whole wheat
bread
1 tomato
½ Bermuda onion
2 tablespoons nonfat salad
dressing
Black coffee or tea and 8 ounces
water

Afternoon Snack
1 cup air-popped popcorn
1 teaspoon grated Parmesan
cheese

Dinner
1 cup spaghetti
½ cup tomato sauce
3 cups Edita's Fountain of Youth
Salad
2 tablespoons nonfat salad
dressing
Black coffee or tea and 8 ounces
water

Bedtime Snack
1 cup Edita's Fountain of Youth
Fruit Salad

DAY 79

Breakfast
1 bagel
2 teaspoons cream cheese
2 teaspoons all-fruit preserves
Black coffee or tea and 8 ounces
water

Morning Snack
1 cup Edita's Fountain of Youth
Fruit Salad
1 cup nonfat fruit yogurt

Lunch
3 cups Edita's Fountain of Youth
Salad
4 ounces canned salmon
2 tablespoons nonfat salad
dressing
Black coffee or tea and 8 ounces
water

Afternoon Snack
1 cup Edita's Fountain of Youth
    Fruit Salad

Dinner
1 baked potato
1 teaspoon grated Parmesan
    cheese
3 cups Edita's Fountain of Youth
    Salad
2 tablespoons nonfat salad
    dressing
4 cups Edita's Fountain of Youth
    Veggies, steamed
½ cup nonfat plain yogurt
¼ cup salsa
Black coffee or tea and 8 ounces
    water

Bedtime Snack
2 slices low-calorie whole wheat
    bread
2 tablespoons all-fruit preserves

DAY 80

Breakfast
1 cup Total® cereal
½ cup skim milk
1 grapefruit
Black coffee or tea and 8 ounces
    water

Morning Snack
2 rice cakes
2 teaspoons all-fruit preserves

Lunch
2 slices low-calorie whole wheat
    bread
1 tomato
½ Bermuda onion
3 cups Edita's Fountain of Youth
    Salad
2 tablespoons nonfat salad
    dressing
Black coffee or tea and 8 ounces
    water

Afternoon Snack
1 apple
1 ounce low-fat Cheddar cheese

Dinner
3 cups Edita's Fountain of Youth
    Salad
2 tablespoons nonfat salad
    dressing
4 cups Edita's Fountain of Youth
    Veggies, steamed
½ cup nonfat plain yogurt
¼ cup salsa
1 baked potato
Black coffee or tea and 8 ounces
    water

Bedtime Snack
1 cup Edita's Fountain of Youth
    Fruit Salad
1 slice raisin bread

DAY 81

Breakfast
3 buttermilk pancakes
2 tablespoons maple syrup
Black coffee or tea and 8 ounces
water

Morning Snack
½ cup carrots
½ cup celery

Lunch
1 baked potato
½ cup nonfat plain yogurt
¼ cup salsa
Black coffee or tea and 8 ounces
water

Afternoon Snack
1 cup air-popped popcorn
1 teaspoon grated Parmesan
cheese

Dinner
1 ground beef patty, grilled or
broiled
2 cups Edita's Fountain of Youth
Salad
2 tablespoons nonfat salad
dressing
4 cups Edita's Fountain of Youth
Veggies, steamed
Black coffee or tea and 8 ounces
water

Bedtime Snack
1 apple
1 fig cookie

DAY 82

Breakfast
1 cup nonfat fruit yogurt
½ cup Total® cereal
Black coffee or tea and 8 ounces
water

Morning Snack
1 cup Edita's Fountain of Youth
Fruit Salad

Lunch
2 slices low-calorie whole wheat
bread
1 ounce low-fat Cheddar cheese
1 tomato
½ Bermuda onion
2 tablespoons nonfat salad
dressing
Black coffee or tea and 8 ounces
water

Afternoon Snack
½ cantaloupe

Dinner
4 ounces skinless chicken breast,
broiled, baked, or grilled
1 cup stuffing
3 cups Edita's Fountain of Youth
Salad
2 tablespoons nonfat salad
dressing
Black coffee or tea and 8 ounces
water

Bedtime Snack
1 bagel
2 teaspoons all-fruit preserves

DAY 83

Breakfast
½ cantaloupe
2 slices low-calorie whole wheat
   bread
2 teaspoons all-fruit preserves
Black coffee or tea and 8 ounces
   water

Morning Snack
1 grapefruit
1 cup nonfat fruit yogurt

Lunch
1 egg
3 cups Edita's Fountain of Youth
   Salad
2 tablespoons nonfat salad
   dressing
Black coffee or tea and 8 ounces
   water

Afternoon Snack
2 rice cakes
2 teaspoons all-fruit preserves

Dinner
4 cups Edita's Fountain of Youth
   Veggies, steamed
3 cups Edita's Fountain of Youth
   Salad
2 tablespoons nonfat salad
   dressing

1 baked potato
Black coffee or tea and 8 ounces
   water

Bedtime Snack
1 cup Edita's Fountain of Youth
   Fruit Salad

DAY 84

Breakfast
1 cup oatmeal
1 tablespoon brown sugar
1 grapefruit
Black coffee or tea and 8 ounces
   water

Morning Snack
½ cantaloupe

Lunch
1 rice cake
1 cup tomato soup made with
   water
3 cups Edita's Fountain of Youth
   Salad
2 tablespoons nonfat salad
   dressing
Black coffee or tea and 8 ounces
   water

Afternoon Snack
1 cup air-popped popcorn
1 teaspoon grated Parmesan
   cheese

Dinner

4 ounces flounder, broiled, baked, or grilled
1 baked potato
3 cups Edita's Fountain of Youth Salad
2 tablespoons nonfat salad dressing
Black coffee or tea and 8 ounces water

Bedtime Snack

1 cup Total® cereal
½ cup skim milk

DAY 85

Breakfast

2 slices French toast
2 tablespoons maple syrup
Black coffee or tea and 8 ounces water

Morning Snack

1 cup nonfat fruit yogurt

Lunch

1 cup vegetable soup
3 cups Edita's Fountain of Youth Salad
2 tablespoons nonfat salad dressing
Black coffee or tea and 8 ounces water

Afternoon Snack

1 slice low-calorie whole wheat bread
1 tomato

Dinner

4 ounces salmon, broiled, baked, grilled, or poached
1 baked potato
4 cups Edita's Fountain of Youth Veggies, steamed
Black coffee or tea and 8 ounces water

Bedtime Snack

1 cup Edita's Fountain of Youth Fruit Salad

DAY 86

Breakfast

1 English muffin
1 cup nonfat fruit yogurt
Black coffee or tea and 8 ounces water

Morning Snack

1 cup Edita's Fountain of Youth Fruit Salad

Lunch

1 pita bread
1 tomato
½ cucumber
¼ Bermuda onion
¼ cup salsa
Black coffee or tea and 8 ounces water

Afternoon Snack
1 apple
1 cup carrots
1 cup celery

Dinner
1 cup spaghetti
½ cup spaghetti sauce
1 teaspoon grated Parmesan
    cheese
3 cups Edita's Fountain of Youth
    Salad
2 tablespoons nonfat salad
    dressing
Black coffee or tea and 8 ounces
    water

Bedtime Snack
1 slice low-calorie whole wheat
    bread
1 teaspoon all-fruit preserves

DAY 87

Breakfast
1 slice low-calorie whole wheat
    bread
1 teaspoon all-fruit preserves
1 cup Edita's Fountain of Youth
    Fruit Salad
Black coffee or tea and 8 ounces
    water

Morning Snack
1 cup vegetable juice
2 rice cakes

Lunch
1 bagel
1 tablespoon cream cheese
2 ounces smoked salmon
1 tomato
½ Bermuda onion, sliced
Black coffee or tea and 8 ounces
water

Afternoon Snack
1 cup nonfat fruit yogurt

Dinner
4 cups Edita's Fountain of Youth
    Veggies, steamed
½ cup plain nonfat yogurt
¼ cup salsa
3 cups Edita's Fountain of Youth
    Salad
2 tablespoons nonfat salad
    dressing
Black coffee or tea and 8 ounces
    water

Bedtime Snack
1 cup Edita's Fountain of Youth
    Fruit Salad
1 fig cookie

DAY 88

Breakfast
1 cup strawberries
1 cup nonfat fruit yogurt
½ cup raisin bran
Black coffee or tea and 8 ounces
    water

Morning Snack
2 rice cakes
2 teaspoons all-fruit preserves

Lunch
2 slices low-calorie whole wheat
  bread
1 ounce low-fat Cheddar cheese
3 cups Edita's Fountain of Youth
  Salad
2 tablespoons nonfat salad
  dressing
Black coffee or tea and 8 ounces
  water

Afternoon Snack
½ cantaloupe

Dinner
4 ounces flounder, broiled, baked,
  or grilled
1 sweet potato, baked
3 cups Edita's Fountain of Youth
  Salad
2 tablespoons nonfat salad
  dressing
Black coffee or tea and 8 ounces
  water

Bedtime Snack
1 slice low-calorie whole wheat
  bread
1 teaspoon all-fruit preserves
1 cup skim milk

DAY 89

Breakfast
1 bagel
1 teaspoon all-fruit preserves
Black coffee or tea and 8 ounces
  water

Morning Snack
½ cantaloupe

Lunch
4 ounces tuna (packed in water)
3 cups Edita's Fountain of Youth
  Salad
2 tablespoons nonfat salad
  dressing
Black coffee or tea and 8 ounces
  water

Afternoon Snack
1 cup Edita's Fountain of Youth
  Fruit Salad

Dinner
1 baked potato
4 cups Edita's Fountain of Youth
  Veggies, steamed
1 cup plain yogurt
½ cup salsa
3 cups Edita's Fountain of Youth
  Salad
2 tablespoons nonfat salad
  dressing
Black coffee or tea and 8 ounces
  water

Bedtime Snack
1 slice low-calorie whole wheat
  bread
1 teaspoon honey
1 cup skim milk

DAY 90

Breakfast
3 blueberry pancakes
2 tablespoons maple syrup
Black coffee or tea and 8 ounces
  water

Morning Snack
1 apple
2 rice cakes

Lunch
1 pita bread
1 tomato
¼ Bermuda onion
3 cups Edita's Fountain of Youth
  Salad

2 tablespoons nonfat salad
  dressing
Black coffee or tea and 8 ounces
  water

Afternoon Snack
1 cup air-popped popcorn
1 teaspoon grated Parmesan
  cheese

Dinner
4 ounces skinless chicken breast,
  broiled, baked, or grilled
1 baked potato
3 cups Edita's Fountain of Youth
  Salad
2 tablespoons nonfat salad
  dressing
Black coffee or tea and 8 ounces
  water

Bedtime Snack
1 slice raisin bread
1 cup Edita's Fountain of Youth
  Fruit Salad

CONGRATULATIONS!

You did it! I'm proud of you. I'll bet you're proud of you too.

Now go back and redo your biological age tests and see just how much younger and thinner you are than you were ninety days ago.

And then come right back, because next comes the wonderful section that will show you how to get even younger and thinner, if you like, or how to stay as slender, vital, and youthful as you are right now!

PART FOUR

YOUNG AND THIN
FOR A LIFETIME

CHAPTER 11

Fountain of Youth for Life:
The Maintenance Program

Perfection is attained by slow degrees; it requires the hand of time.

—VOLTAIRE

FOUNTAIN OF YOUTH GRADUATE SCHOOL

Congratulations! You've graduated. You are younger than you were just a short ninety days ago. You are thinner (I hope you've treated yourself to a terrific new outfit) than you were ninety days ago—thinner than you have been for a very long time. You are healthier than you were ninety days ago. In ninety short days you have improved your chances for reaching your maximum life span. That's great! Imagine what you can achieve in the next ninety days, and the next, and the next . . . So don't lose that momentum. Don't lose those extra precious years, that slender youthful figure, and that healthy bod. Keep it up. Keep it going. Get to 100! Get to 120!

Every graduate deserves a graduation present. Here's yours—a maintenance program that will keep you younger, thinner, and healthier, a program that gives you your own personal fountain of youth for life!

SUPERSTARS: 125 FOUNTAIN OF YOUTH FOODS

Here are the top anti-aging foods you will need for your lifetime program. There's nothing stingy about this list: loads and loads of choices, low in fat, high in goodness, no counting, no measuring, just enjoyment. Sounds good to me. Fresh, frozen, and even canned, these are the foods richest in antioxidants, dense with anti-aging and weight-loss magic. These are the foods that will be part of your *Fountain of Youth* for life.

Apples
Apple juice, unsweetened
Applesauce, unsweetened
Apricots, fresh and dried
Arugula
Asparagus
Bagels
Bananas
Barley
Beans, all kinds
Beet greens
Beets
Bell peppers, green, red, and
  yellow
Blackberries
Blueberries
Bok choy
Boysenberries
Bran cereal
Bread, raisin
Bread, rye
Bread stuffing
Bread, white and whole wheat
Broccoli
Brussels sprouts
Bulgur wheat
Butter Buds®
Buttermilk
Cabbage, red and white
Cantaloupe
Carrots

Cauliflower
Celery
Cheese, low-fat
Cherries
Chicken breast
Chicken broth
Chickpeas
Chili peppers
Chives
Clams
Collard greens
Cookies, fig
Corn
Couscous
Cranberries
Cranberry juice
Cream of wheat
Cucumber
Currants
Dandelion greens
Dill weed
Eggplant
Eggs
Egg substitute
Endive
English muffins
Figs
Fish
Flour tortilla
Fortune cookies
Fruit salad, in juice

Garlic
Gingersnap cookies
Grapefruit
Grapefruit juice
Grapes
Green beans
Grits
Kale
Leeks
Lettuce, all kinds
Mango
Melons, all kinds
Milk, skim
Mineral water
Mushrooms
Mustard greens
Oat bran
Oatmeal
Okra
Onions
Oranges
Orange juice
Pancakes
Papaya
Parsley
Pasta
Peaches
Pears
Peas
Pineapple
Pineapple juice
Pita bread

Popcorn, air-popped
Potato
Preserves, all-fruit
Prune juice
Prunes
Pumpkin
Pumpkin seeds
Radish
Raisins
Rice cakes
Salad dressing, nonfat
Salmon, canned
Sardines, canned
Spinach
Squash
Strawberries
Sweet potatoes
Swiss chard
Taco shells
Tea
Tofu
Tomatoes
Tomato juice
Tuna, canned in water
Turkey breast
Turnip
Turnip greens
Vegetable juice
Watermelon
Yogurt, all kinds, low-fat
    or nonfat
Zucchini

TAKING OFF THE TRAINING WHEELS

Remember when you were little and you could hardly wait to take off those training wheels and fly on your two-wheeler like the big kids? Guess what? Now that your ninety days are over, the training wheels come off right now. You are ready to develop anti-aging and weight-loss food plans for yourself. Here are some good choices to get you started. When you feel a little more confident, you will be able to make instant anti-aging and weight-loss selections. In fact, nothing else will appeal to the younger thinner you.

Build a Meal of Your Own: Breakfast Choices

Bagels
Bread
Oatmeal
Cream of wheat
Waffles
Pancakes
English muffins
Bran cereal

Breakfast "go withs"
Brown sugar
All-fruit preserves
Maple syrup
Cream cheese, low-fat or nonfat

Build a Meal of Your Own: Lunches

Water-packed tuna
Canned sardines in tomato sauce
Canned salmon
Egg substitute or eggs
Cheeses, low-fat or nonfat
Bagels
Pita bread
Taco shells
Salads with nonfat salad dressing
Deli meats like sliced chicken, ham, or turkey, nonfat
Soups made with water or skim milk
Sliced tomatoes, onions, and cucumbers
Cream cheese, nonfat

Build a Meal of Your Own: Snacks

Fruits or fruit salad in juice
Yogurt, fruit-flavored, low-fat or nonfat
Breads or crackers, low-fat
Bagels
Juice, fruit or vegetable
Popcorn, air-popped with Parmesan cheese
Fig cookies or gingersnaps
Cereals
Raisins and other dried fruit

Build a Meal of Your Own: Dinners

4 ounces skinless chicken breast, baked, broiled, or grilled
4 ounces skinless turkey breast, baked, broiled, or grilled
1 hamburger patty, grilled
3 ounces low-fat beef, broiled or grilled
Pasta with vegetables or clam sauce
Steamed vegetables
Tossed salad with nonfat salad dressing
Egg substitute or eggs
Tofu
Fish, broiled, baked, or grilled
Soups made with water or skim milk
Sweet potatoes or regular potatoes
Assorted herbs and spices
Butter Buds®
Salsa

THE KISS FORMULA

KISS=Keep It Simply Simple

Whether you are shopping, cooking, eating out, or ordering in, the *Fountain of Youth* is simple to live. Here are some tips to help you always follow the KISS formula.

YOUR FIRST KISS: STOCKING THE PERFECT <u>FOUNTAIN OF YOUTH</u> KITCHEN

Hate shopping? I don't blame you. I used to hate it too. I felt like I needed a calculator to figure out the fat, the calories, the daily allowances. I thought they were supposed to make labels easier. I felt like a dummy. Finally, frustrated, stressed out, and often just plain hungry, I stopped caring what went into my shopping cart and what I brought into my kitchen. But all that was before *Fountain of Youth*. Now, shopping is a breeze. In fact, I love to go. I can zip through the grocery store in no time flat. My grocery bill is easily 20 percent or more lower than it used to be. I can shop with half a brain while the other decides on what wonderful new, skinny outfit I'm going to indulge my new, wonderful skinny body with. This can be you, too. Come on, let's go grocery shopping. It's easy.

EDITA'S THREE GROCERY SHOPPING RULES
Shop the rim first—that's where most of the anti-aging goodies are.
Always buy nonfat—that's where the skinny comes in.
Stick with the list—that's where the healthy is.

The Master Grocery List

Water, bottled, mineral, plain, or bubbly
Diet soda
Cheese, nonfat, any kind
Yogurt, plain and fruit flavored, nonfat
Milk, skim and reinforced with calcium
Milk, evaporated skim
Milk, dry nonfat
Eggs
Egg substitute

Coffee, regular and decaf
Tea, regular, decaf, and herbal
Pancake mix, low-fat
Frozen waffles, low-fat
Maple syrup, reduced-fat and/or -calorie
Preserves, all-fruit
Salsa
Rice cakes, assorted flavors
Popcorn for air popping
Tuna, canned, packed in water
Tofu
Salmon, canned
Sardines, canned, packed in water or tomato sauce
Spaghetti sauce, low-fat
Juice, unsweetened, fortified with vitamins or calcium
Parmesan cheese, grated, low-fat
Beans, assorted, dried or canned
Olive, canola, or safflower oil
Vegetable cooking spray
Canned soups, low-fat, low-sodium, assorted
Dried soups, assorted
Canned chicken broth, low-sodium
Canned vegetables, assorted
Canned fruit, assorted, packed in its own juice
Fresh fruit, assorted
Dried fruit, assorted
Fresh vegetables, assorted
Frozen vegetables, assorted
Greens, dark green, assorted
Sweet potatoes, regular potatoes
Deli sliced ham, turkey, or chicken, nonfat
Fresh skinless chicken breast
Fresh turkey
Ground lean beef, turkey, and veal
Fresh veal
Fresh fish
Nonfat salad dressing, assorted
Herbs and spices, assorted
Pasta, any and all kinds
Bread, bagels, pita

Rice, white and brown
Cookies (fig, gingersnaps, fortune, and graham and animal crackers)
Cake, angel food
Frozen yogurt, nonfat
Fruit juice bars
Bran cereal such as Total®

There, now you're done. Fast, simple, and no labels to struggle over and interpret. No stress, no fuss, no mistakes. Everything in your shopping basket and in your kitchen is there to keep you getting younger and thinner with every meal.

For the Doubting Thomases

I know that some of you out there are feeling pretty good about the wonderful changes you're seeing and feeling, both inside and out. You are full of energy, bursting with vitality. Your blood pressure, heart rate, cholesterol, and other indicators of premature aging are all lower. And best of all your closet is filled with some very exciting fashions in some very exciting sizes. This is not the time to get cocky. If you stick with the *Fountain of Youth* foods and the shopping list you'll be fine—better than fine. If you don't you might just find yourself smack dab in a big mess of aging fat.

But there comes a moment when every *Fountain of Youth* graduate wants to "go it on their own." Here's what I've heard: "Edita, I don't need really tight, proscribed lists of foods." Or, "I'm not going to make any shopping mistakes, I know what to buy." Or—this is my favorite— "Edita, after ninety days and the wonderful new me, do you really think I'm going to buy something that is loaded with fat?" This last one usually comes with rolling eyeballs and that "I'm smarter than the teacher" look. So go ahead. Try throwing something into your shopping cart that's not on the list. But before you do take this little test.

The Fat Label Test

Opposite is a typical food label. How much fat are we really talking about? I'm going to make it really easy. This is as far as you need to read on any label.

A SAMPLE LABEL: MACARONI & CHEESE

Standardized ———

Nutrition Facts

Serving Size: ½ cup
Servings Per Container: 4

Amount Per Serving   — *New*

Calories 260   Calories from Fat 120   — *New*

	% Daily Value *
Total Fat 13 g	**20**%
Saturated Fat 5 g	**25**%
Cholesterol 30 mg	**10**%
Sodium 660 mg	**28**%
Total Carbohydrate 31 g	**11**%
Dietary Fiber 0 g	**0**%
Sugars 5 g	
Protein 5 g	

New ‹

Vitamin A 4% • Vitamin C 2% • Calcium15% • Iron 4%

* Percents (%) of a Daily Value are based on a
2,000 calorie diet. Your Daily Values may vary
higher or lower depending on your calorie needs:

Nutrient		2,000 Calories	2,500 Calories
Total Fat		Less than	65 g	80 g
Sat. Fat	Less than	20 g	25 g
Cholesterol	Less than	300 mg	300 mg
Sodium	Less than	2,400 mg	2,400 mg
Total Carbohydrate		300 g	375 g
Fiber		25 g	30 g

— *New*

1g Fat = 9 calories
1g Carbohydrate = 4 calories
1g Protein = 4 calories

New ———

1. What percentage of the total calories are fat?_____
Nutrition Facts
Serving Size: ½ cup
Servings Per Container: 4
Amount Per Serving
Calories 260
Calories from Fat 120
Total Fat 13 g

2. Here's another one. (Imagine the label.)
What percentage of total calories are fat?_____
Nutrition Facts
Serving Size: ¾ cup
Servings Per Container: 11
Amount Per Serving
Calories 110
Calories from Fat 10
Total Fat 1 g

3. Here's one more. (Imagine the label.)
What percentage of total calories are fat?_____
Nutrition Facts
Serving Size: 1 can
Servings Per Container: 3
Amount Per Serving
Calories 80
Calories from Fat 10
Total Fat 1 g

4. Okay, last one, I promise. (Imagine the label.)
What percentage of total calories are fat?_____
Nutrition Facts
Serving Size: ½ cup
Servings Per Container: 6
Amount Per Serving
Calories 100
Calories from Fat 45
Total Fat 5 g

Answers
1. 45%—a definite no-no
2. 8%—great
3. 11%—good
4. 45%—another no-no (See how tricky it is, even though it says only
   100 calories and just 5 grams of fat.)

If you didn't get a perfect score, stick to the list. Even though labels have been redesigned and reconfigured, they are still a major fat trap for even the most sophisticated *Fountain of Youth* shoppers.

FOOD CALCULATIONS AND COMPUTATIONS

RDAs

RDAs (Recommended Dietary Allowances) are minimal requirements of various nutrients necessary to prevent disease in healthy people.

Portions and Servings

3 ounces of cooked fish or chicken is about the size of a deck of cards.
1 medium apple is the size of a tennis ball.
1 ounce of cheese is the size of four dice or a large marble.
½ cup broccoli is the size of a lightbulb.
1 teaspoon jam is the size of 4 stacked quarters.
1 slice of bread is the size of a cassette tape.
½ cup salad or pasta is the size of the inside of half a tennis ball.
1 average muffin is the size of a baseball.
½ cup serving of cooked rice will fit into a teacup.

Calorie Requirements

It takes 1 calorie per minute to keep your basic metabolism going. That's about 1,500 calories in any one 24-hour period.
   One pound of fat contains 3,500 calories.

Figuring Fat

Daily Calories	Fat in grams		
	20%	25%	30%
1,200	27	33	40
1,400	31	39	47
1,600	36	44	53
1,800	40	50	60
2,000	44	56	67
2,200	49	61	73

How Much Fat in Something?

Grams of fat x 9 x 100 = fat intake
Total calories

HOW TO FIGURE YOUR MINIMUM FIVE FRUIT AND VEGETABLE SERVINGS

1 Vegetable Serving
- 1 cup raw leafy vegetables, including endive, escarole, romaine, spinach, or other salad greens
- ½ cup other vegetables, such as carrots, cauliflower, green beans, peppers, leeks, and cabbage
- ¾ cup vegetable juice
- 1 medium tomato
- 5 asparagus spears
- 1 medium stalk broccoli

1 Fruit Serving
- 1 medium apple, banana, orange, or peach
- 2 medium plums or tangerines
- ⅓ cantaloupe
- ⅛ honeydew melon
- 15 small grapes
- ½ cup cut-up raw, cooked, or canned fruit
- 8 medium strawberries
- ¾ cup blueberries

Food Tips
- Making packaged rice and sauce? Skip the butter.
- Making stuffing? Skip the butter.
- Order small sizes of snacks, burgers, and shakes.
- Don't eat croutons on your salad. Substitute a couple of crackers.
- Use nonstick pans or a little vegetable cooking spray instead of oil.
- Switch to nonfat cheeses—no fat, same calcium.
- Switch to skim milk—no fat, same calcium.
- Throw out fatty condiments like tartar sauce, mayo, and others.
- Steam your scallops.

- Cream cheese is a better bet than butter.
- Forget peanut butter and have the jelly.
- Add slices of nonfat cheese to your sandwiches.
- Have a salad with every meal: fruit salad with breakfast, green salad with lunch and dinner.
- Flavor your water with lemon or lime juice.
- Have grilled cheese with tomato, not bacon.
- Switch to lite syrup.
- Start using liquid egg substitute.
- Make tuna and chicken sandwiches with plain nonfat yogurt.
- Crunch celery with your sandwich, instead of chips.
- Buy nonfat cold cuts from your deli counter.
- Try fresh tomatoes, garlic, and basil on your pasta instead of prepared tomato sauces.
- Top chicken potpie with mashed potatoes, not piecrust.
- Eat more fish.
- Switch to bagels for breakfast.
- Buy low-fat bread—it's great and you can have an extra slice.
- Use low-sodium canned veggies.
- Experiment with flavored decaf coffees for an after-dinner treat.
- Add tofu to a recipe for a new taste treat.
- Try making some oriental recipes with oriental ingredients.
- Blot your slice of pizza and leave off the meat.
- Keep a bowl of cut-up veggies in your fridge for fast snacks.
- Keep a bowl of cut-up fruit in your fridge for fast snacks.
- Look for new products reinforced with vitamins and calcium.
- Invest in a popcorn popper and forget the microwave.
- Have a hard mint or toffee-type candy to satisfy your sugar craving.
- Sometimes frozen veggies can have more nutrients than fresh because they are flash frozen and don't have to travel to your grocer's shelf.

HERE'S YOUR SECOND KISS: COOKING YOUNGER, COOKING THINNER

Now that you've come back from the grocery store with loads of youth-making goodies, don't blow it between the stove and the table. Just as shopping young and thin is easy, cooking young and thin is easy too. Just follow the formula.

As God Is My Witness, I'll Never Fry Again

Frying is out—deep, shallow, whatever. You will never fry again. That's all you need to know about frying.

Sauté the Fountain of Youth Way

This is one of the basic ways to fix fantastic *Fountain of Youth* foods. There are only two ways you are going to sauté, with ¼ cup of chicken stock, vegetable stock, water, or white wine or with a light *poof* of cooking spray.

Grilling All Year Round

Chicken, turkey, low-fat burgers, fish, veggies, whatever—it all works on the grill. Line the grill with foil and skewer the ingredients. Grill. Or season, wrap in foil, and a few minutes later, dinner is served with no fat, all the nutrients, and no pots or pans to wash.

Veggie	Grilling Time for Veggies Cut In Chunks
Corn	25 minutes
Eggplant	10 minutes
Fennel	15 minutes
Garlic	30 minutes
Leeks	12 minutes
Mushrooms	8 minutes
Onions	20 minutes
Peppers	12 minutes
Potatoes	10 minutes
Squash	10 minutes
Tomatoes	10 minutes

Stir-Fry Comes Out of the Oriental Closet

All you need is a big wok or skillet, a little liquid, finely chopped veggies, a smidgen of meat or fish, a dash of seasoning, and dinner is served. It looks great, it's fun to make, and it's filled with anti-aging goodness.

Fondue: The Next Generation

Remember fondue? Sure you do, we all did it in the sixties. A candle, cheap wine, and a pot filled with oil bubbling away. Wonderful. Now welcome to the fondue of the future. Same pot, but bubbling with chicken broth. Cook bits of chicken, veal, or fish. And some veggies. What do you have? A wonderful revival that's fun, social, and healthy. Go on. Dig out that old fondue pot. It's probably somewhere in the attic. You'll be glad you did.

Get Steamed

Whether you chose your microwave or a large pot with a steamer, this is one of the best ways to fix veggies. A dash of seasonings, a splash of nonfat salad dressing, a side bowl of salsa-spiked yogurt and you've got a fast, fabulous, *Fountain of Youth* meal.

> Research finds that lightly steaming vegetables, like carrots, releases more anti-aging beta-carotene.

Spice It Up

There are more spices in the world of the young and thin than salt. So get rid of that salt shaker and get creative. When you go shopping buy one new spice every week and experiment. After six weeks, you won't even miss the salt. Do the same with herbs. Many grocery stores sell fresh herbs in little pots. Buy a couple and put them on your kitchen window or counter. They look great, taste even better, and many, like parsley, rosemary, and basil, pack a powerful antioxidant punch all on their own.

HERE'S YOUR THIRD KISS: FIX YOUR FAVORITES THE <u>FOUNTAIN OF YOUTH</u> WAY

Your Morning Coffee

Using a paper filter essentially eliminates the cholesterol-raising compounds in coffee. This doesn't mean you can drink coffee all day long, but when you fix it, use a good filter or switch to decaf. Never stir artificial creamer into your coffee. Go for a teaspoon or two of dry powdered skim milk or a shot of bottled skim milk. You'll add calcium and cut out the fat.

Your Favorites Fixed the <u>Fountain of Youth</u> Way

Pull out your favorite recipe. Now list all the no-no ingredients on this chart, including preparation methods. Next, go to the *Fountain of Youth* Now-You-See-It, Now-You-Don't Substitutions and fix your favorites the *Fountain of Youth* way.

Ingredients	Amounts	Changes
_____	_____	_____
_____	_____	_____
_____	_____	_____
_____	_____	_____
_____	_____	_____
_____	_____	_____
_____	_____	_____

Preparation Method	Changes
_____	_____
_____	_____
_____	_____
_____	_____
_____	_____
_____	_____

When Ingredients Call for:	Switch to:
whole eggs	2 egg whites or egg substitute
whole milk	skim milk
sugar	½ cup sugar per cup of flour in cakes
	1 tablespoon sugar per cup of flour in yeast breads
baking chocolate, 1 ounce	3 tablespoons cocoa
fat	baby food fruit purees or applesauce for all the fat
heavy cream	evaporated skim milk
sour cream	plain nonfat yogurt

More Negative Fat Tricks for Family Favorites

Macaroni and cheese: Switch to skim milk, cut the fat in half or more, and skip the salt.

Bread stuffing: Skip the added fat. Use chicken broth and extra seasoning.

Scalloped and au gratin spuds: Cut the fat by half or more. Use skim milk and low-fat or nonfat cheese.

Thicker soups and gravies: Use instant mashed potatoes.

THE MINEFIELDS

It would be easy to follow the *Fountain of Youth* if you were locked in a padded cell and wonderful food trays were slipped under your door six times a day. But you don't. You live, work, function, and eat in the real world. And the real world is filled with *Fountain of Youth* minefields. There are fast-food places on every corner, donuts snuggle up to morning bagels, fries call your name seductively. So what's a person to do?

I. Think Thin, Think Young

It took you a very long time to get prematurely old and fat. The *Fountain of Youth* is a miracle program but it isn't *Bewitched* where you twitch and the result is instant. Don't get frustrated. Don't be impatient. Just count off the days—one at a time.

2. Stay Away from Alcohol

I know—all the studies say that a glass of wine cuts your risk of heart disease. True. But wait until you get to the weight and age you want before you have that glass of wine a day. Why? Because other studies show that drinking alcoholic beverages leads to a caloric intake far beyond what your body needs. First of all, alcohol has empty calories of its own, and second, it triggers cravings for protein and fats.

3. The Work Traps

For the duration of the *Fountain of Youth* program try to be antisocial. Stay away from the coffee wagon, the lunchroom, the candy and soda machines, the inevitable birthday, anniversary, or retirement party. A better bet is to pack your own lunch and snacks and get out of the building for those all-important walks. If you have a buddy at work who is also on the *Fountain of Youth* program, great! The two of you can reinforce each other while you both get younger and thinner every day.

4. Eating Out

Can't avoid dinner or brunch out? Simply take your daily *Fountain of Youth* program page with you and eat as though you were at home. Go for veggies, salads, breads, and fruit. And don't tell me that there isn't a restaurant in this country where you can't get something from the menu that fits the *Fountain of Youth* day you are on. You can. I did.

5. The Family Saboteurs

Mothers, mates, and kids are the number one *Fountain of Youth* busters. Yes, you love them all. No, you aren't going to stuff your face with fat, age-making foods to prove it. Just smile and say no.

Help! I'm Stuck

This is a tough one. Your body is a living, breathing, reacting, sensitive piece of wonder. It is not anything like the thermostat on an air conditioner. You turn it down and down it goes. You are not going to lose a pound every single day. You may get stuck. You may not lose a single pound for two days, three days, even a week or more. You may even gain a pound or two. Normal. All this is perfectly normal. That doesn't mean nothing is happening. You are losing weight—your scale just hasn't registered the fact yet. You are getting younger—the clock is turning back with every bite. Do not panic. Do not weep with frustration. Do not eat an entire pint of ice cream. Do not give up. Stay with it. You'll see.

> Even if the scale seems stuck, the calendar isn't. You are getting younger every day.

How to Get UnStuck

- Take an extra walk.
- Don't stop eating required foods.
- Drink an extra glass or two of water.
- Buy something that fits whatever number of pounds you have lost.
- Don't think about it.
- Believe.

NOW THAT YOU ARE TRULY ON YOUR OWN

I have just a few last-minute instructions to share with you. Please take them to heart.

1. **The Rule of Five: Eat at least five servings of fruits and veggies every day.**
2. **Nutrient- and antioxidant-dense wins every time.**
3. **Drink your water, juice, and herbal tea.**
4. **Life isn't dull. Your meals shouldn't be either. Get variety. Experiment.**

Go ahead, enjoy!

FAST-TRACK AGE BUSTER AND WEIGHT-LOSS PROGRAM

Impatient? Excited? Psyched? Motivated? Big Date?

This fast-track program will reverse your clock and melt those pounds faster. You will see results after just thirty days. Take the tests on day 1. Compare your results after the fast-track program to your starting numbers. Then continue for another sixty days on the regular *Fountain of Youth* program.

Here's What You Do

√ Take the same tests you would take if you were starting the regular *Fountain of Youth* program. Write down your results.
√ Go shopping to make sure you have all the ingredients and foods you will need. Use the handy weekly shopping lists.
√ Pick a low-stress time to start this fast-track program.
√ Curtail your socializing and restaurant hopping for thirty days.

The fast-track <u>Fountain of Youth</u> program is designed for thirty days. After thirty days go back to the regular program for sixty days.

DAY 1

Breakfast
1 cup Total® cereal
½ cup skim milk
Black coffee or tea and 8 ounces
    water
10-minute walk

Morning Snack
½ cantaloupe
10-minute walk

Lunch
1 slice low-calorie whole wheat
    bread

1 tomato
3 cups Edita's Fountain of Youth
    Salad
2 tablespoons nonfat salad
    dressing
Black coffee or tea and 8 ounces
    water
10-minute walk

Afternoon Snack
1 cup nonfat fruit yogurt
10-minute walk

Dinner
3 ounces skinless chicken breast,
    baked, broiled, or grilled

4 cups Edita's Fountain of Youth
   Veggies, steamed
2 tablespoons nonfat salad
   dressing
Black coffee or tea and
   8 ounces water
10-minute walk

Bedtime Snack
1 slice low-calorie whole wheat
   bread
1 teaspoon all-fruit preserves
Herbal tea
10-minute walk

DAY 2

Breakfast
1 bagel
1 teaspoon all-fruit preserves
Black coffee or tea and 8 ounces
   water
10-minute walk

Morning Snack
1 cup Edita's Fountain of Youth
   Fruit Salad
10-minute walk

Lunch
4 ounces tuna (packed in water)
3 cups Edita's Fountain of Youth
   Salad
2 tablespoons nonfat salad
   dressing
Black coffee or tea and 8 ounces
   water
10-minute walk

Afternoon Snack
1 low-fat fruit yogurt
10-minute walk

Dinner
1 baked potato
4 cups Edita's Fountain of Youth
   Veggies, steamed
3 cups Edita's Fountain of Youth
   salad
½ cup nonfat plain yogurt
¼ cup salsa
Black coffee or tea and 8 ounces
   water
10-minute walk

Bedtime Snack
1 slice low-calorie whole wheat
   bread
1 teaspoon all-fruit preserves
Herbal tea
10-minute walk

DAY 3

Breakfast
1 English muffin
1 teaspoon all-fruit preserves
Black coffee or tea and 8 ounces
   water
10-minute walk

Morning Snack
½ cup carrots
½ cup plain nonfat yogurt
¼ cup salsa
10-minute walk

Lunch
1 slice low-calorie whole wheat
  bread
1 hard-boiled egg
3 cups Edita's Fountain of Youth
  Salad
2 tablespoons nonfat salad
  dressing
Black coffee or tea and 8 ounces
  water
10-minute walk

Afternoon Snack
1 cup nonfat fruit yogurt
10-minute walk

Dinner
3 ounces white meat turkey,
  baked, broiled, or grilled
1 cup brussels sprouts, steamed
1 sweet potato, baked
2 tablespoons nonfat dressing
Black coffee or tea and 8 ounces
  water
10-minute walk

Bedtime Snack
1 rice cake
1 teaspoon honey
Herbal tea
10-minute walk

DAY 4

Breakfast
1 cup oatmeal
1 tablespoon brown sugar

Black coffee or tea and 8 ounces
  water
10-minute walk

Morning Snack
½ cantaloupe
10-minute walk

Lunch
1 rice cake, any flavor
1 cup tomato soup made with
  water
3 cups Edita's Fountain of Youth
  Salad
2 tablespoons nonfat salad
  dressing
Black coffee or tea and 8 ounces
  water
10-minute walk

Afternoon Snack
1 cup air-popped popcorn
1 teaspoon grated Parmesan
  cheese
10-minute walk

Dinner
4 ounces flounder, broiled
1 sweet potato, baked
3 cups Edita's Fountain of Youth
  Salad
2 tablespoons nonfat salad
  dressing
Black coffee or tea and 8 ounces
  water
10-minute walk

Bedtime Snack

1 cup bran cereal
½ cup skim milk
Herbal tea
10-minute walk

DAY 5

Breakfast

1 slice low-calorie whole wheat
    bread
1 teaspoon all-fruit preserves
Black coffee or tea and 8 ounces
    water
10-minute walk

Morning Snack

1 cup vegetable juice
10-minute walk

Lunch

1 bagel
1 teaspoon nonfat cream cheese
1 tomato, sliced
1 slice onion
Black coffee or tea and 8 ounces
    water
10-minute walk

Afternoon Snack

1 cup nonfat fruit yogurt
10-minute walk

Dinner

1 baked potato
4 cups Edita's Fountain of Youth
    Veggies, steamed

¼ cup salsa
3 cups Edita's Fountain of Youth
    Salad
2 tablespoons nonfat salad
    dressing
Black coffee or tea and 8 ounces
    water
10-minute walk

Bedtime Snack

1 cup Edita's Fountain of Youth
    Fruit Salad
10-minute walk

DAY 6

Breakfast

1 cup strawberries
1 cup nonfat fruit yogurt
Black coffee or tea and 8 ounces
    water
10-minute walk

Morning Snack

1 rice cake
1 teaspoon all-fruit preserves
10-minute walk

Lunch

1 slice low-calorie whole wheat
    bread
1 slice (1 ounce) nonfat Cheddar
    or Swiss cheese
3 cups Edita's Fountain of Youth
    Salad
2 tablespoons nonfat salad
    dressing

Black coffee or tea and 8 ounces
    water
10-minute walk

Afternoon Snack
½ cup cantaloupe
10-minute walk

Dinner
1 cup cooked spaghetti
½ cup spaghetti sauce
1 teaspoon grated Parmesan
    cheese
3 cups Edita's Fountain of Youth
    Salad
2 tablespoons nonfat salad
    dressing
Black coffee or tea and 8 ounces
    water
10-minute walk

Bedtime Snack
1 slice low-calorie whole wheat
    bread
1 teaspoon all-fruit preserves
Herbal tea
10-minute walk

DAY 7

Breakfast
3 blueberry pancakes
2 tablespoons maple syrup
Black coffee or tea and 8 ounces
    water
10-minute walk

Morning Snack
1 orange
10-minute walk

Lunch
1 pita bread
1 tomato, cut into chunks
¼ onion, cut into chunks
1 ounce shredded nonfat Cheddar
    or other cheese
¼ cup salsa
½ cup shredded lettuce
Black coffee or tea and 8 ounces
    water
10-minute walk

Afternoon Snack
1 cup air-popped popcorn
1 teaspoon grated Parmesan
    cheese
10-minute walk

Dinner
4 cups Edita's Fountain of Youth
    Veggies, steamed
1 baked potato
2 tablespoons nonfat salad
    dressing
Black coffee or tea and 8 ounces
    water
10-minute walk

Bedtime Snack
½ cantaloupe
10-minute walk

DAY 8

Breakfast
1 bagel
1 teaspoon all-fruit preserves
Black coffee or tea and 8 ounces
    water
10-minute walk

Morning Snack
1 cup nonfat fruit yogurt
10-minute walk

Lunch
4 ounces tuna (packed in water)
3 cups Edita's Fountain of Youth
    Salad
2 tablespoons nonfat salad
    dressing
Black coffee or tea and 8 ounces
    water
10-minute walk

Afternoon Snack
1 apple
10-minute walk

Dinner
3 ounces skinless chicken breast,
    baked, broiled, or grilled
1 sweet potato, baked
4 cups Edita's Fountain of Youth
    Veggies, steamed
½ cup plain nonfat yogurt
¼ cup salsa
Black coffee or tea and 8 ounces
    water
10-minute walk

Bedtime Snack
1 cup bran cereal
½ cup skim milk
Herbal tea
10-minute walk

DAY 9

Breakfast
1 English muffin
1 teaspoon all-fruit preserves
1 cup nonfat fruit yogurt
Black coffee or tea and 8 ounces
    water
10-minute walk

Morning Snack
½ cantaloupe
10-minute walk

Lunch
1 cup vegetable soup made with
    water
2 rice cakes
2 teaspoons nonfat cream cheese
1 tomato, sliced
Black coffee or tea and 8 ounces
    water
10-minute walk

Afternoon Snack
1 cup air-popped popcorn
1 teaspoon grated Parmesan
    cheese
10-minute walk

Dinner

1 baked potato
1 teaspoon grated Parmesan
   cheese
4 cups Edita's Fountain of Youth
   Veggies, steamed
2 tablespoons nonfat salad
   dressing
Black coffee or tea and 8 ounces
   water
10-minute walk

Bedtime Snack

1 slice low-calorie whole wheat
   bread
1 teaspoon all-fruit preserves
Herbal tea
10-minute walk

DAY 10

Breakfast

1 cup oatmeal
1 tablespoon brown sugar
Black coffee or tea and 8 ounces
   water
10-minute walk

Morning Snack

1 cup nonfat fruit yogurt
10-minute walk

Lunch

1 cup tomato soup made with
   water
2 rice cakes
3 cups Edita's Fountain of Youth
   Salad

2 tablespoons nonfat salad
   dressing
Black coffee or tea and 8 ounces
   water
10-minute walk

Afternoon Snack

1 cup strawberries
10-minute walk

Dinner

4 ounces salmon, baked, broiled,
   or poached
1 baked potato
4 cups Edita's Fountain of Youth
   Veggies, steamed
2 tablespoons nonfat salad
   dressing
Black coffee or tea and 8 ounces
   water
10-minute walk

Bedtime Snack

1 cup Edita's Fountain of Youth
   Fruit Salad
Herbal tea
10-minute walk

DAY 11

Breakfast

1 cup Total® cereal
½ cup skim milk
Black coffee or tea and 8 ounces
   water
10-minute walk

Morning Snack
1 cup nonfat fruit yogurt
10-minute walk

Lunch
2 ounces skinless turkey breast,
    sliced
1 slice low-calorie whole wheat
    bread
1 teaspoon cream cheese
1 tomato, sliced
Black coffee or tea and 8 ounces
    water
10-minute walk

Afternoon Snack
1 apple
10-minute walk

Dinner
1 cup spaghetti
½ cup spaghetti sauce
1 teaspoon grated Parmesan
    cheese
3 cups Edita's Fountain of Youth
    Salad
2 tablespoons nonfat salad
    dressing
Black coffee or tea and 8 ounces
    water
10-minute walk

Bedtime Snack
1 slice low-calorie whole wheat
    bread
1 teaspoon all-fruit preserves
Herbal tea
10-minute walk

DAY 12

Breakfast
1 cup nonfat fruit yogurt
½ cup raisin bran cereal
Black coffee or tea and 8 ounces
    water
10-minute walk

Morning Snack
½ cup carrots
½ cup red pepper
10-minute walk

Lunch
1 cup vegetable soup made with
    water
1 rice cake
10-minute walk

Afternoon Snack
1 cup Edita's Fountain of Youth
    Fruit Salad
10-minute walk

Dinner
3 ounces skinless turkey breast,
    baked, broiled, or grilled
4 cups Edita's Fountain of Youth
    Veggies, steamed
2 tablespoons nonfat salad
    dressing
Black coffee or tea and 8 ounces
    water
10-minute walk

Bedtime Snack
1 slice low-calorie whole wheat
    bread
1 teaspoon honey
Herbal tea
10-minute walk

DAY 13

Breakfast
2 slices French toast
2 tablespoons maple syrup
Black coffee or tea and 8 ounces
    water
10-minute walk

Morning Snack
1 orange
10-minute walk

Lunch
4 ounces tuna (packed in water)
3 cups Edita's Fountain of Youth
    Salad
2 tablespoons nonfat salad
    dressing
Black coffee or tea and 8 ounces
    water
10-minute walk

Afternoon Snack
1 cup air-popped popcorn
1 tablespoon grated Parmesan
    cheese
10-minute walk

Dinner
4 ounces flounder, baked or
    broiled
4 cups Edita's Fountain of Youth
    Veggies, steamed
2 tablespoons nonfat salad
    dressing
Black coffee or tea and 8 ounces
    water
10-minute walk

Bedtime Snack
1 slice low-calorie whole wheat
    bread
1 teaspoon all-fruit preserves
Herbal tea
10-minute walk

DAY 14

Breakfast
1 bagel
1 teaspoon all-fruit preserves
Black coffee or tea and 8 ounces
    water
10-minute walk

Morning Snack
1 cup vegetable juice
1 rice cake
10-minute walk

Lunch
1 hamburger patty, grilled
3 cups Edita's Fountain of Youth
    Salad
2 tablespoons nonfat salad
    dressing

Black coffee or tea and 8 ounces
water
10-minute walk

Afternoon Snack
½ cantaloupe
10-minute walk

Dinner
4 cups Edita's Fountain of Youth
Veggies, steamed
1 baked potato
½ cup plain nonfat yogurt
¼ cup salsa
Black coffee or tea and 8 ounces
water
10-minute walk

Bedtime Snack
1 cup skim milk
1 slice raisin bread
10-minute walk

Day 15

Breakfast
1 cup Total® cereal
½ cup skim milk
Black coffee or tea and 8 ounces
water
10-minute walk

Morning Snack
½ cantaloupe
10-minute walk

Lunch
1 slice low-calorie whole wheat
bread
1 tomato, sliced
3 cups Edita's Fountain of Youth
Salad
2 tablespoons nonfat salad
dressing
Black coffee or tea and 8 ounces
water
10-minute walk

Afternoon Snack
1 cup nonfat fruit yogurt
10-minute walk

Dinner
3 ounces skinless chicken breast,
baked, broiled, or grilled
4 cups Edita's Fountain of Youth
Veggies, steamed
2 tablespoons nonfat salad
dressing
Black coffee or tea and 8 ounces
water
10-minute walk

Bedtime Snack
1 slice low-calorie whole wheat
bread
1 teaspoon all-fruit preserves
Herbal tea
10-minute walk

Day 16

Breakfast
1 bagel

1 teaspoon all-fruit preserves
Black coffee or tea and 8 ounces
    water
10-minute walk

Morning Snack
1 cup Edita's Fountain of Youth
    Fruit Salad
10-minute walk

Lunch
4 ounces tuna (packed in water)
3 cups Edita's Fountain of Youth
    Salad
2 tablespoons nonfat salad
    dressing
Black coffee or tea and 8 ounces
    water
10-minute walk

Afternoon Snack
1 cup low-fat fruit yogurt
10-minute walk

Dinner
1 baked potato
4 cups Edita's Fountain of Youth
    Veggies, steamed
3 cups Edita's Fountain of Youth
    Salad
½ cup nonfat plain yogurt
¼ cup salsa
Black coffee or tea and 8 ounces
    water
10-minute walk

Bedtime Snack
1 slice low-calorie whole wheat
    bread
1 teaspoon all-fruit preserves

Herbal tea
10-minute walk

DAY 17

Breakfast
1 English muffin
1 teaspoon all-fruit preserves
Black coffee or tea and 8 ounces
    water
10-minute walk

Morning Snack
½ cup carrots
½ cup plain nonfat yogurt
¼ cup salsa
10-minute walk

Lunch
1 slice low-calorie whole wheat
    bread
1 hard-boiled egg
3 cups Edita's Fountain of Youth
    Salad
2 tablespoons nonfat salad
    dressing
Black coffee or tea and 8 ounces
    water
10-minute walk

Afternoon Snack
1 cup nonfat fruit yogurt
10-minute walk

Dinner
3 ounces white meat turkey,
    baked, broiled, or grilled
1 cup brussels sprouts, steamed

1 sweet potato, baked
2 tablespoons nonfat salad
  dressing
Black coffee or tea and 8 ounces
  water
10-minute walk

Bedtime Snack
1 rice cake
1 teaspoon honey
Herbal tea
10-minute walk

DAY 18

Breakfast
1 cup oatmeal
1 tablespoon brown sugar
Black coffee or tea and 8 ounces
  water
10-minute walk

Morning Snack
½ cantaloupe
10-minute walk

Lunch
1 rice cake, any flavor
1 cup tomato soup made with
  water
3 cups Edita's Fountain of Youth
  Salad
2 tablespoons nonfat salad
  dressing
Black coffee or tea and 8 ounces
  water
10-minute walk

Afternoon Snack
1 cup air-popped popcorn
1 teaspoon grated Parmesan
  cheese
10-minute walk

Dinner
4 ounces flounder, broiled
1 sweet potato, baked
3 cups Edita's Fountain of Youth
  Salad
2 tablespoons nonfat salad
  dressing
Black coffee or tea and 8 ounces
  water
10-minute walk

Bedtime Snack
1 cup bran cereal
½ cup skim milk
Herbal tea
10-minute walk

DAY 19

Breakfast
1 slice low-calorie whole wheat
  bread
1 teaspoon all-fruit preserves
Black coffee or tea and 8 ounces
  water
10-minute walk

Morning Snack
1 cup vegetable juice
10-minute walk

Lunch

1 bagel
1 teaspoon nonfat cream cheese
1 tomato, sliced
1 slice onion
Black coffee or tea and 8 ounces
    water
10-minute walk

Afternoon Snack

1 cup nonfat fruit yogurt
10-minute walk

Dinner

1 baked potato
4 cups Edita's Fountain of Youth
    Veggies, steamed
¼ cup salsa
3 cups Edita's Fountain of Youth
    Salad
2 tablespoons nonfat salad
    dressing
Black coffee or tea and 8 ounces
    water
10-minute walk

Bedtime Snack

1 cup Edita's Fountain of Youth
    Fruit Salad
10-minute walk

DAY 20

Breakfast

1 cup strawberries
1 cup nonfat fruit yogurt
Black coffee or tea and 8 ounces
    water
10-minute walk

Morning Snack

1 rice cake
1 teaspoon all-fruit preserves
10-minute walk

Lunch

1 slice low-calorie whole wheat
    bread
1 slice (1 ounce) nonfat Cheddar
    or Swiss cheese
3 cups Edita's Fountain of Youth
    Salad
2 tablespoons nonfat salad
    dressing
Black coffee or tea and 8 ounces
    water
10-minute walk

Afternoon Snack

½ cantaloupe
10-minute walk

Dinner

1 cup cooked spaghetti
½ cup spaghetti sauce
1 teaspoon grated Parmesan
    cheese
3 cups Edita's Fountain of Youth
    Salad
2 tablespoons nonfat salad
    dressing
Black coffee or tea and 8 ounces
    water
10-minute walk

Bedtime Snack

1 slice low-calorie whole wheat
    bread
1 teaspoon all-fruit preserves
Herbal tea
10-minute walk

DAY 21

Breakfast
3 blueberry pancakes
2 tablespoons maple syrup
Black coffee or tea and 8 ounces
    water
10-minute walk

Morning Snack
1 orange
10-minute walk

Lunch
1 pita bread
1 tomato, cut into chunks
¼ onion, cut into chunks
1 ounce shredded nonfat Cheddar
    or other cheese
¼ cup salsa
½ cup shredded lettuce
Black coffee or tea and 8 ounces
    water
10-minute walk

Afternoon Snack
1 cup air-popped popcorn
1 teaspoon grated Parmesan
    cheese
10-minute walk

Dinner
4 cups Edita's Fountain of Youth
    Veggies, steamed
1 baked potato
2 tablespoons nonfat salad
    dressing

Black coffee or tea and 8 ounces
    water
10-minute walk

Bedtime Snack
½ cantaloupe
10-minute walk

DAY 22

Breakfast
1 bagel
1 teaspoon all-fruit preserves
Black coffee or tea and 8 ounces
    water
10-minute walk

Morning Snack
1 cup nonfat fruit yogurt
10-minute walk

Lunch
4 ounces tuna (packed in water)
3 cups Edita's Fountain of Youth
    Salad
2 tablespoons nonfat salad
    dressing
Black coffee or tea and 8 ounces w
    water
10-minute walk

Afternoon Snack
1 apple
10-minute walk

Dinner
3 ounces skinless chicken breast,
    baked, broiled, or grilled

1 sweet potato, baked
4 cups Edita's Fountain of Youth
    Veggies, steamed
½ cup plain nonfat yogurt
¼ cup salsa
Black coffee or tea and 8 ounces
    water
10-minute walk

Bedtime Snack
1 cup bran cereal
½ cup skim milk
Herbal tea
10-minute walk

Day 23

Breakfast
1 English muffin
1 teaspoon all-fruit preserves
1 cup nonfat fruit yogurt
Black coffee or tea and 8 ounces
    water
10-minute walk

Morning Snack
½ cantaloupe
10-minute walk

Lunch
1 cup vegetable soup made with
    water
2 rice cakes
2 teaspoons nonfat cream cheese
1 tomato, sliced
Black coffee or tea and 8 ounces
    water
10-minute walk

Afternoon Snack
1 cup air-popped popcorn
1 teaspoon grated Parmesan
    cheese
10-minute walk

Dinner
1 baked potato
1 teaspoon grated Parmesan
    cheese
4 cups Edita's Fountain of Youth
    Veggies, steamed
2 tablespoons nonfat salad
    dressing
Black coffee or tea and 8 ounces
    water
10-minute walk

Bedtime Snack
1 slice low-calorie whole wheat
    bread
1 teaspoon all-fruit preserves
Herbal tea
10-minute walk

Day 24

Breakfast
1 cup oatmeal
1 tablespoon brown sugar
Black coffee or tea and 8 ounces
    water
10-minute walk

Morning Snack
1 cup nonfat fruit yogurt
10-minute walk

Lunch

1 cup tomato soup made with
  water
2 rice cakes
3 cups Edita's Fountain of Youth
  Salad
2 tablespoons nonfat salad
  dressing
Black coffee or tea and 8 ounces
  water
10-minute walk

Afternoon Snack

1 cup strawberries
10-minute walk

Dinner

4 ounces salmon, baked, broiled,
  or poached
1 baked potato
4 cups Edita's Fountain of Youth
  Veggies, steamed
2 tablespoons nonfat salad
  dressing
Black coffee or tea and 8 ounces
  water
10-minute walk

Bedtime Snack

1 cup Edita's Fountain of Youth
  Fruit Salad
Herbal tea
10-minute walk

DAY 25

Breakfast

1 cup Total® cereal
½ cup skim milk

Black coffee or tea and 8 ounces
  water
10-minute walk

Morning Snack

1 cup nonfat fruit yogurt
10-minute walk

Lunch

2 ounces skinless turkey breast,
  sliced
1 slice low-calorie whole wheat
  bread
1 teaspoon cream cheese
1 slice tomato
Black coffee or tea and 8 ounces
  water
10-minute walk

Afternoon Snack

1 apple
10-minute walk

Dinner

1 cup spaghetti
½ cup spaghetti sauce
1 teaspoon grated Parmesan
  cheese
3 cups Edita's Fountain of Youth
  Salad
2 tablespoons nonfat salad
  dressing
Black coffee or tea and 8 ounces
  water
10-minute walk

Bedtime Snack

1 slice low-calorie whole wheat
  bread
1 teaspoon all-fruit preserves

Herbal tea
10-minute walk

DAY 26

Breakfast
1 cup nonfat fruit yogurt
½ cup raisin bran cereal
Black coffee or tea and 8 ounces
    water
10-minute walk

Morning Snack
½ cup carrots
½ cup red pepper
10-minute walk

Lunch
1 cup vegetable soup made with
    water
1 rice cake
10-minute walk

Afternoon Snack
1 cup Edita's Fountain of Youth
    Fruit Salad
10-minute walk

Dinner
3 ounces skinless turkey breast,
    baked, broiled, or grilled
4 cups Edita's Fountain of Youth
    Veggies, steamed

2 tablespoons nonfat salad
    dressing
Black coffee or tea and 8 ounces
    water
10-minute walk

Bedtime Snack
1 slice low-calorie whole wheat
    bread
1 teaspoon honey
Herbal tea
10-minute walk

DAY 27

Breakfast
2 slices French toast
2 tablespoons maple syrup
Black coffee or tea and 8 ounces
    water
10-minute walk

Morning Snack
1 orange
10-minute walk

Lunch
4 ounces tuna (packed in water)
3 cups Edita's Fountain of Youth
    Salad
2 tablespoons nonfat salad
    dressing
Black coffee or tea and 8 ounces
    water
10-minute walk

Afternoon Snack

1 cup air-popped popcorn
1 tablespoon grated Parmesan
   cheese
10-minute walk

Dinner

4 ounces flounder, baked or
   broiled
4 cups Edita's Fountain of Youth
   Veggies, steamed
2 tablespoons nonfat salad
   dressing
Black coffee or tea and 8 ounces
   water
10-minute walk

Bedtime Snack

1 slice low-calorie whole wheat
   bread
1 teaspoon all-fruit preserves
Herbal tea
10-minute walk

Day 28

Breakfast

2 slices French toast
2 tablespoons maple syrup
Black coffee or tea and 8 ounces
   water
10-minute walk

Morning Snack

1 orange
10-minute walk

Lunch

4 ounces tuna (packed in water)
3 cups Edita's Fountain of Youth
   Salad
2 tablespoons nonfat salad
   dressing
Black coffee or tea and 8 ounces
   water
10-minute walk

Afternoon Snack

1 cup air-popped popcorn
1 tablespoon grated Parmesan
   cheese
10-minute walk

Dinner

4 ounces flounder, baked or
   broiled
4 cups Edita's Fountain of Youth
   Veggies, steamed
2 tablespoons nonfat salad
   dressing
Black coffee or tea and 8 ounces
   water
10-minute walk

Bedtime Snack

1 slice low-calorie whole wheat
   bread
1 teaspoon all-fruit preserves
Herbal tea
10-minute walk

DAY 29

Breakfast
1 bagel
1 teaspoon all-fruit preserves
Black coffee or tea and 8 ounces
    water
10-minute walk

Morning Snack
1 cup vegetable juice
1 rice cake
10-minute walk

Lunch
1 hamburger patty, grilled
3 cups Edita's Fountain of Youth
    Salad
2 tablespoons nonfat salad
    dressing
Black coffee or tea and 8 ounces
    water
10-minute walk

Afternoon Snack
½ cup cantaloupe
10-minute walk

Dinner
4 cups Edita's Fountain of Youth
    Veggies, steamed
1 baked potato
½ cup plain nonfat yogurt
¼ cup salsa
Black coffee or tea and 8 ounces
    water
10-minute walk

Bedtime Snack
1 cup skim milk
1 slice raisin bread
10-minute walk

DAY 30

Breakfast
1 cup Total® cereal
½ cup skim milk
Black coffee or tea and 8 ounces
    water
10-minute walk

Morning Snack
1 rice cake
1 teaspoon all-fruit preserves
10-minute walk

Lunch
1 pita bread
1 tomato, chopped
½ cup chopped lettuce
2 tablespoons salsa
Black coffee or tea and 8 ounces
    water
10-minute walk

Afternoon Snack
1 cup nonfat fruit yogurt
10-minute walk

Dinner
4 ounces salmon, baked, broiled,
    or poached
4 cups Edita's Fountain of Youth
    Veggies, steamed
1 baked potato
2 tablespoons nonfat salad
    dressing

Black coffee or tea and 8 ounces
   water
10-minute walk

Bedtime Snack
½ cantaloupe
10-minute walk

CHAPTER 12

The Fountain of Youth Lifestyle

Where there's a will, there's a way.

—ENGLISH PROVERB

THE <u>FOUNTAIN OF YOUTH</u> LIFE

You've probably already figured this out. The *Fountain of Youth* isn't just for ninety days. This is the way to live, and live, and live for 43,800 days—that's 1 million hours, that's the whole 120 years! The ninety days you just went through was just to get you to start loving broccoli, your great skin, fantastic checkups, and that alive feeling when you fasten your two- or three- or six-sizes-smaller pants.

And even though this is a book about food, longevity, and weight loss it wouldn't be complete without a few words about other facts that impact on our longevity and our weight to a greater or lesser degree. So, here goes.

THE GRANDPARENTS MYTH BLOWN

No, it isn't true that if your grandparents lived to a ripe old age, you will too. At least it's only partly true and you may be surprised by how very small the part really is. According to studies, genetics and lifestyle play a somewhat balanced role in your health—that is, until you really begin to age. Then the way you have lived your life rather than the genes you may have inherited becomes the critical factor. Abuse your health and even grandparents who lived to 100 won't be able to save you from a premature death.

In the past twenty years the study of genetics has unlocked some remarkable secrets. Specific locations in our genetic blueprint have been found for diabetes, muscular dystrophy, and cystic fibrosis. Statistical evidence is coming to light that points to a genetic component or predisposition to obesity; high blood pressure; colon, lung, and breast cancers; alcoholism; schizophrenia; and Alzheimer's disease. But scientists have not been able to really find a genetic link to longevity. However, since there are over 1 billion letters in the DNA code strung along forty-six chromosomes providing space for 100,000 genes, there may still be one gene that determines how long our family history gives us to live. If such a longevity gene is there, we haven't found it yet, and until we do, you better eat your broccoli.

Long-lived grandparents have only a 15 to 20 percent effect on your own longevity. The rest is how well you live.

The same goes for fat. Saying that fat runs in your family just isn't going to fly anymore. Even though scientists have strong suspicions that obesity may be genetic to some extent, they maintain that even if you have a genetic tendency to be fat, you yourself have a great deal of control over whether your fat genes dominate your life, or whether you remain slender and fit and overcome your fat genetics.

DESTRESS

There is absolutely no doubt: Stress is aging, fattening, and can kill you. It also triggers off a massive free radical feeding frenzy that can batter you so severely inside that you never recover. I'm not just talking about the occasional stress. You know when you are pulled over for a broken taillight and you get those guilty sweats, or when you get excited at the basketball championships, or when you win the lottery. All those good and bad experiences are short-term stress responses. After you pull away with a promise to get that light fixed, after your team wins or loses, and after you invest your lottery winnings, your stress response goes back to normal. You calm down. And so do the free radicals.

Killer stress is the stress response that never stops. This is the stress junkie kind of stress, the kind that always needs that stress high, that adrenaline fix. Well, that adrenaline fix if left to pour out into your system is toxic. It floods your cells and, if unrelieved, can overwhelm your body's defenses to deal with it. Part of the *Fountain of Youth* lifestyle is to modulate your responses to stress so that you have balance between times of calm and times of intensity.

Studies show that antioxidants can reduce much of the damage caused by excessive stress, but not all of it. Find ways of dealing with your stress that are healthy: counseling, stress management courses, hobbies, a change of lifestyle, whatever. If you get a handle on your stress you will be helping antioxidants do their life-restoring job.

SMOKING

I can't believe I'm even writing about smoking. All I can say is, if you smoke, stop. In case you missed it, one of the major stimulants of free radicals is cigarette smoke. It isn't enough that your body produces plenty of free radicals just by breathing; it really isn't necessary to add to the free radicals you already have by inhaling them from the exhaust of cigarettes. Use whatever works. Just stop. And then start eating carrots to reduce your risk of developing lung cancer.

ALCOHOL

There is enough evidence to suggest that a glass of red wine or an alcoholic beverage can help reduce your risk of a heart attack. There is also enough evidence to show that purple grape juice does the same thing. If you have not changed your eating habits or your lifestyle, all the red wine in the world isn't going to protect you. Some alcohol may very well be medicinal, but on the downside alcohol stimulates the appetite, so we tend to overeat and eat the wrong things when we drink.

Here's another option: Change your diet to include loads of antioxidants, get some exercise every day, and then revisit the alcohol issue.

A GOOD MIND-SET

Scientists have isolated several personality characteristics among those who age successfully—stay healthy, look good, have energy, and do exciting things into their seventies, eighties, and nineties. And one of the main factors is a positive mind-set, a feeling of control over one's self and one's life. They are optimists who love to laugh. It's called "getting a life" and it's never too late or too soon to start.

A good mind-set works wonders for weight loss, too.

EXERCISE

What can I say about exercise except that it is like an extra antioxidant. Right after the Olympics the U.S. Centers for Disease Control and Prevention released the first ever *Surgeon General's Report on Physical Activity and Health.* Designed to give a swift kick in the pants to couch potatoes, just like other Surgeon Generals' reports changed smokers into nonsmokers and got everyone to buckle up, this report intends to get America off the couch and moving.

Not only is lack of activity fattening, it's deadly. There are enough studies that show a lack of activity and exercise increases the risk of premature death, cardiovascular disease, colon cancer, heart attack, high blood pressure, osteoporosis, and more. The Cooper Institute of Aerobics Research in Dallas found in a recent study that the risk of dying prematurely if you are sedentary is the same as if you smoked a pack of cigarettes a day. The study went on to say that sitting around is an even more serious health risk than high blood pressure, high cholesterol, obesity, or family history of diabetes.

Still sitting on that couch? Here are some more studies that should scare you into your first walk.

- USC School of Medicine reports that women who exercise three or more hours per week can lower their risk of breast cancer by 30 percent at age forty.
- Studies reported in *Medicine and Science in Sports and Exercise* show that getting regular exercise helps to retard the decline in immune function that so often is one of the first signs of aging and triggers diseases that lead to premature death.

- Exercise can offer better odds to smokers. A new study in the *Journal of the American Medical Association* found that physically fit smokers had lower death rates than nonsmokers who were out of shape. This doesn't mean that it's okay to smoke. What it does mean is that if you smoke, improved fitness may increase your life expectancy and even out the odds of negative life expectancy factors.
- Fitness offers protection against the aging effects of stress and can lower blood pressure, according to a study at Duke University Medical Center.
- An ongoing Harvard study found that those people who burned 2,000 or more calories per week through exercise had a 28 percent lower death rate than those who didn't. How much exercise burns 2,000 calories a week? It depends on your weight and on the intensity, but a sixty-minute walk burns off about 300 calories. So walking every day should do it.
- Exercise offers protection against the development of colon cancer.
- A recent study published in the *Journal of Aging and Physical Activity* found that walking can keep your brain sharp by improving blood flow.

WEIGHTS

Starting as early as thirty you lose 6½ pounds of muscle every ten years. So what? So with muscle loss, your metabolism slows down about 2 percent every ten years and so you burn less and gain more. Your bones start to thin around the same time at a rate of 5 percent annually in the first ten years following menopause. How to rejuvenate? Weights.

YOUNGER SKIN

Smoking, stress, sun all add years to your skin. Alpha Hydroxy Acids (AHAs) helped reduce the visible signs of aging skin. Now Beta Hydroxy is the next generation of skin care. The result? Younger, fresher-looking skin.

THE <u>FOUNTAIN OF YOUTH</u> EXERCISE PLAN

I'm not going to give you any fancy charts on how many calories you can burn by going to the fridge and back or how many calories you can burn dusting off your treadmill. Forget that. If you want to get the maximum benefit from your antioxidants, if you want to get thinner, get younger, and live longer there is one thing you need to do. It's easy. It's fast. It's cheap. It's portable. It's nonnegotiable. And it's an integral part of the *Fountain of Youth.*

Walk for 30 to 60 minutes a day.

I big walk of 60 minutes
or
2 smaller walks of 30 minutes
or
4 short walks of 15 minutes
or
6 mini walks of 10 minutes
or
12 itty bitty walks of 5 minutes
or
It doesn't matter. Just do it.

CHAPTER 13

Welcome to the Future

If you think you can, you can.
And if you think you can't, you're right.

—MARY KAY ASH

MIRROR, MIRROR ON THE WALL, WHO'S THE YOUNGEST (AND THINNEST) OF THEM ALL?

Silly question. You are, of course. And you are going to stay that way, aren't you? Sure you are. Because the alternative—fat, sick, old, and dead—is just not acceptable anymore.

And you know how to keep that young, slender, healthy body you've just created. You know that long-lived grandparents give you a small edge, but that how you live, what you eat, how much you exercise, how well you manage stress, how little you smoke and drink and abuse your body is far, far more important to staying younger for longer.

Now we've almost completed this part of our journey together. I'm very proud of you. You are a winner. But before we leave each other let's just take a peek into the future. Aren't you curious to see just what scientists are working on to help us stay young, thin, and healthy to that million-hour max—the 120-year human life span potential? I am.

NEW LIFE EXTENSION RESEARCH

Human Growth Hormone

No, this doesn't work on the principle that if you're taller you can weigh more. Nice try, though. Human growth hormone is produced in the pituitary gland and its main job, which it does during the night shift, is to regulate our growth. So, as you have already figured out, its biggest job is from the time we are born until we stop growing. But our reaching full maturity doesn't mean this little hormone doesn't keep right on pumping. It does. And with every single spurt, it reduces body fat and increases the amount of lean mass of muscle, bone, and other organs.

In a well-publicized experiment a group of elderly men were given injections of human growth hormone and guess what? Their spare tires, love handles, and flab were replaced with young, vigorous, lean muscle tissue.

Keep your eye on this one. It may be a future answer to hormonal liposuction, exercise, and dieting all rolled into one.

Melatonin: A Miracle in Longevity?

There are a slew of books out there on this formerly shy and obscure hormone, now thrust into the anti-aging limelight. So, is this really the new longevity treatment? Can it reverse human aging? Stimulate libido? Win the war against cancer and AIDS? Boost immunity? Can it really stop heart attacks, Sudden Infant Death Syndrome, depression, and whatever else you can name? The jury is still out. So far what melatonin can do is help with jet lag, shift work, and sleep by resetting the body's clock. Whether melatonin can also affect the timer that goes off when we're done living is yet to be seen. But stick around. This one shows some real promise.

Genetic Engineering

This is the Erector set of anti-aging research. Geneticists are working feverishly to manipulate the one gene that monitors and regulates human aging. If they can fiddle with the mechanism of the death gene, scientists believe they can extend the human life span indefinitely. Experiments in the lab are beginning to show some real progress. And experiments in genetic engineering with other life forms are pointing the way to human studies. But this life extension solution is still in the realm of sci-fi, so don't stop eating your carrots and broccoli just yet.

DHEA: The Fat Burner Plus

Even though hardly anyone outside a lab can even pronounce it, dehydroepiandrosterone, an experimental adrenal steroid known as DHEA for short, is another new member of the futuristic anti-aging team.

This one started with a very chubby dog named Duchess from Wisconsin. Duchess was spayed and, as is often the case, she gained a lot of weight after the procedure. Duchess was eight years old and waddled along, dragging with her fatty deposits in her belly, sides, and haunches. Sound familiar?

Then a team of vets injected Duchess with DHEA and the weight literally melted off her. No matter what she ate, she lost weight. Why? DHEA is a kind of fat thermostat. It regulates the conversion of carbohydrates to fat so that extra carbs don't get stored as fat; they get burned off as energy.

That was about ten years ago. In the intervening years scientists have found evidence that DHEA lowers cholesterol, especially the "bad" LDL kind in animals by 30 percent. Animals getting DHEA also lowered their risk of cancers, seemed to be able to rejuvenate tired organs, and had a much healthier immune system.

What about humans? Scientists know that this is the most abundant steroid hormone in our bodies. It's been around since the early 1930s. About ten years ago, interest began because scientists noticed that there is a drop-off in DHEA after we reach twenty-five. They asked themselves whether this drop-off in DHEA has something to do with bodies getting older. If we were able to keep DHEA levels high, could we push back the physical signs of aging? Could we stop the onset and progress of aging diseases like heart disease and cancer? So far, preliminary studies are looking pretty good. Women with breast cancer, for example, seem to have less DHEA than women without breast cancer. The same goes for heart attack victims.

So far much of the evidence on humans is still to come but that hasn't stopped over seven thousand physicians around the country from writing prescriptions for DHEA and health food stores and vitamin specialty shops from keeping a good stock on hand.

The Starvation Solution

This sounds like it shouldn't work, the idea being the less we eat, the fewer calories we consume, the longer we live. Called caloric restriction or chronic energy intake restriction, it's one of the more serious contenders in the anti-aging wars.

Experiments conducted on laboratory rats found those whose daily calories were severely restricted lived almost 50 percent longer and were healthy, vigorous, and had a great sex life. (It's possible that they had more time for sex because they spent less time eating.)

But—and this is a big *but*—the diets of these rats, even though they were fed 70 percent fewer calories, still had foods that were nutrient dense and their diets were supplemented with vitamins and other rat nutrients.

Researchers found that this caloric restriction also delayed the onset of cancers, kidney failure, and immune-system decline normally associated with aging tissues. The underfed rats also had lower blood pressure and less incidence of diabetes, and appeared to handle stress very well. Their systems, flooded with antioxidant-rich nutrients and not clogged up with free radical—causing fats and other substances, appeared to be rejuvenated.

Similar benefits seem possible for humans who choose this as one of the ways they will fight off the inevitability of age, disease, and metabolic decline.

The Last Word

And now we have come, not to the end of our journey together, but to a new beginning. Keep it up. Enjoy. Be healthy. Be happy. Live long and prosper.

PART FIVE

FOUNTAIN OF
YOUTH
COOKBOOK

SPOONABLE FRENCH TOAST

Makes 1 serving

2 slices of cinnamon raisin bread
Egg substitute to equal 1 egg
1 cup skim milk
1 teaspoon maple syrup
Dash of cinnamon
Cooking spray

Cut the raisin bread in ½-inch cubes. In a small bowl using a whisk, mix together the egg substitute, milk, maple syrup, and cinnamon. Throw the cubes of bread into the mixture and toss to make sure they are evenly coated. Pour the mixture into a small nonstick skillet coated lightly with cooking spray. Cook on medium, stirring, until the mixture is set.

YOUTH NUTRIENTS PER SERVING

Calories	456
Calcium	474 mg
Vitamin C	3 mg
Beta-carotene	5,922 IU

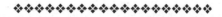

MAKE THE SWITCH TO SKIM

A study from the University of Minnesota School of Public Health found that switching from whole milk to skim milk lowered cholesterol levels by 7 percent in just six weeks.

ESPRESSO WAKE-UP SHAKE

Makes 1 serving

¾ cup skim milk
1 banana
2 teaspoons instant coffee dissolved in ¼ cup orange juice
2 tablespoons frozen orange juice concentrate
Dash of nutmeg

Combine the milk, banana, coffee with orange juice, and orange juice concentrate in a blender or food processor and process until smooth. Top with a dash of nutmeg.

YOUTH NUTRIENTS PER SERVING

Calories	226
Calcium	245 mg
Vitamin C	61 mg
Beta-carotene	565 IU

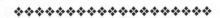

HOME IS WHERE THE CAFFEINE IS

According to a reader survey in <u>Income Opportunities</u> magazine, 79 percent of work-at-home business folks skip breakfast while 65 percent want coffee and want it with caffeine.

THE PALM BREAKFAST SHAKE

Makes 2 servings

½ cup skim milk
½ cup plain low-fat yogurt
½ cup strawberries
½ cup papaya chunks
3 to 4 large ice cubes

Combine the milk, yogurt, strawberries, and papaya in a blender. Cover and blend until smooth. Add the ice cubes, one at a time, blending after each addition. Pour into fancy glasses and serve.

YOUTH NUTRIENTS PER SERVING

Calories	82
Calcium	193 mg
Vitamin C	44 mg
Beta-carotene	272 IU

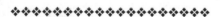

A+ FOR PAPAYA

One cup of papaya gives you lots of vitamin C and is a great change from oranges.

BREAKFAST DESSERT PARFAIT

Makes 4 servings

1 banana, sliced
1 cup kiwifruit, peeled and sliced
1 cup strawberries, washed, hulled, and sliced
1 cup vanilla low-fat yogurt
1 cup Total® cereal

In a small bowl, mix the banana, kiwi, and strawberries together. Put a layer of fruit, a layer of yogurt, and a layer of cereal into 4 parfait glasses. Serve at once.

YOUTH NUTRIENTS PER SERVING

Calories	130
Calcium	198 mg
Vitamin C	97 mg
Beta-carotene	142 IU

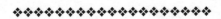

THE SNIFF AND LOSE TEST

Researchers at the Smell and Taste Treatment and Research Foundation in Chicago found that subjects who sniffed a blend of banana, peppermint, and green apples; had a well-developed sense of smell; and ate a sensible diet lost nearly thirty pounds in six months. It seems the brain can be fooled into thinking sniffing is swallowing.

POWER BREAKFAST BARS

Makes 24 servings

Cooking spray
4 cups Total® cereal
1 cup raisins
½ cup dried figs, chopped into small pieces
½ cup dried apricots, chopped into small pieces
¼ cup margarine
2 cups cut-up marshmallows

Lightly spray a 13 x 9-inch baking pan with cooking spray.

In a large bowl, mix together the cereal, raisins, figs, and apricots. Set aside.

In a medium saucepan on medium heat, melt the margarine. Add the marshmallows and cook until they melt. Stir often.

Pour the melted marshmallow mixture into the fruit mixture and mix until all the fruit is coated with the marshmallow mixture.

Using the back of a plastic spoon or your hands, press the mixture into the baking pan, spreading it evenly.

Chill for an hour. Cut into 24 bars. You can store these bars in airtight containers for a week.

Youth Nutrients Per Serving

Calories	76
Calcium	53 mg
Vitamin C	10 mg
Beta-carotene	399 IU

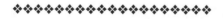

GET ON THE "BRAN WAGON"

A study from the Arizona Cancer Center found that adding bran and calcium to your diet can reduce your risk of developing colon cancer.

HOT AND COLD FRUIT BREAKFAST BOWL

Makes 4 servings

6 ounces dried fruit mix
1 cup orange juice
¼ cup water
¼ cup sugar
2 cups vanilla frozen yogurt

In a medium saucepan, heat the dried fruit mix, orange juice, water, and sugar to boiling. Reduce the heat. Cover and simmer for about 30 minutes, or until the dried fruit mix is tender. Divide the frozen yogurt among 4 pretty dessert dishes. Spoon the hot fruit mixture on top.

YOUTH NUTRIENTS PER SERVING

Calories	294
Calcium	126 mg
Vitamin C	33 mg
Beta-carotene	1,315 IU

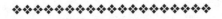

OLD SAYING

The only difference between a rut and a grave is the depth.

SWEET BREAKFAST MOUTHFULS

Makes 24 mouthfuls

3 egg whites
⅔ cup sugar
4 cups Total® cereal
½ cup raisins

Preheat the oven to 325°F.

In a medium bowl, using a hand mixer or whisk, beat the egg whites until they are foamy. Add the sugar, a little at a time, beating after each addition. Mix in the cereal and the raisins and stir gently until the cereal is coated. Drop by spoonfuls on a nonstick cookie sheet. Bake for 14 to 16 minutes.

YOUTH NUTRIENTS PER SERVING

Calories	49
Calcium	43 mg
Vitamin C	10 mg
Beta-carotene	1 IU

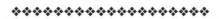

A LITTLE DIET HUMOR

The second day of a diet is always easier than the first—by the second day you're off of it.

MMMM MUFFINS

Makes 12 servings

1½ cups canned pumpkin pie filling
4 egg whites
½ cup skim milk
1 teaspoon vanilla extract
1 teaspoon cinnamon
1 teaspoon nutmeg
2 cups biscuit mix
½ cup raisins

Preheat the oven to 350°F.

In a large bowl, mix together the pumpkin pie filling, egg whites, and milk until well mixed; then add the rest of the ingredients. Fill 12 paper muffin cups set into metal muffin tins with equal amounts of the batter. Bake for 20 minutes, or until a toothpick inserted into the center comes out clean.

YOUTH NUTRIENTS PER SERVING

Calories	143
Calcium	57 mg
Vitamin C	2 mg
Beta-carotene	2,822 IU

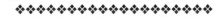

A LITTLE MORE DIET HUMOR

What is dieting? Tightening the belt on your birthday suit.

BANANA SPLIT BREAKFAST

Makes 4 servings

1 kiwifruit, peeled and chopped
1 orange, peeled and chopped
1 cup strawberries, hulled and quartered
2 bananas, peeled and split lengthwise
1 cup vanilla low-fat yogurt
Cinnamon

In a medium bowl, mix together the kiwifruit, orange, and strawberries. On each of 4 salad plates, place one half of a banana. Top with ¼ cup yogurt. Sprinkle ¼ of the fruit mixture on top and finish off with a dusting of cinnamon. Serve at once.

YOUTH NUTRIENTS PER SERVING

Calories	142
Calcium	128 mg
Vitamin C	66 mg
Beta-carotene	193 IU

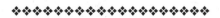

THE LAW OF BALANCE

Bad habits will cancel out good ones. For example, the orange juice and granola you had for breakfast will be canceled out by the cigarette you smoked on the way to work and the candy bar you just bought.

HANS CHRISTIAN ANDERSEN MUESLI

Makes 2 servings

1 cup instant rolled oats
1 cup plain low-fat yogurt
1 apple, peeled and shredded
¼ cup raisins

In medium bowl, mix all the ingredients together. Place the muesli in an airtight container and refrigerate overnight. When you are ready for breakfast divide the mixture into bowls and enjoy.

YOUTH NUTRIENTS PER SERVING

Calories	314
Calcium	261 mg
Vitamin C	6 mg
Beta-carotene	87 IU

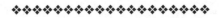

ROLLED OATS TIPS

Add a handful of rolled oats instead of bread crumbs to ground hamburger. Make a hot bowl of oatmeal for a bedtime snack. Whip up a batch of oatmeal and raisin cookies (low-fat, of course) for a sweet treat that's good for you.

JUICY SHAKE

Makes 4 servings

2 cups vanilla nonfat yogurt
6 ounces frozen orange juice concentrate
1 cup orange slices

Put all the ingredients in a blender or food processor and process until smooth. Pour into glasses and serve at once.

YOUTH NUTRIENTS PER SERVING

Calories	192
Calcium	234 mg
Vitamin C	83 mg
Beta-carotene	216 IU

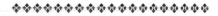

JUICY ALTERNATIVES

Try juicing fresh apples, apricots, handfuls of berries, fresh grapefruit, grapes, mangoes, melons, nectarines, papayas, peaches, pineapple, and tangerines. Make up your own antioxidant combos.

SWEET POTATO PANCAKES

Makes 8 servings

2 sweet potatoes, peeled and shredded
¼ cup all-purpose flour
1 cup liquid egg substitute
1 onion, peeled and grated
Cooking spray
8 tablespoons plain low-fat or nonfat yogurt
8 tablespoons unsweetened applesauce
¼ teaspoon nutmeg

Put the shredded potatoes on a double thickness of paper towel and pat dry to get some of the moisture out of them. In a medium bowl, combine the flour, shredded potatoes, egg substitute, and onion. Mix until well blended.

Spray a large skillet with cooking spray and place over medium-high heat. For each pancake spoon about ¼ cup of mixture onto the hot skillet. Spread it out into a circle with the back of a long-handled spoon. Cook for about 5 minutes and turn. Cook again for about 5 minutes, or until golden. Remove the first batch and keep warm. Repeat until all the batter is used up.

Serve hot with a spoonful of yogurt and applesauce dusted with nutmeg.

YOUTH NUTRIENTS PER SERVING

Calories	99
Calcium	62 mg
Vitamin C	9 mg
Beta-carotene	7,201 IU

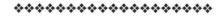

BREAKFAST FOR YOUR BRAIN

New studies show that your brain needs breakfast after a long night without brain food—glucose. Your memory and attention span will be better all day. What's the best choice? A little fruit or juice.

SMOKED SALMON DESIGNER BREAKFAST PIZZA

Makes 6 servings

1 16-ounce package frozen pizza dough, thawed
3 cups shredded low-fat or nonfat mozzarella
1 red onion, sliced thin and separated into rings
2 tomatoes, sliced thin
6 ounces smoked salmon, cut into thin strips
6 teaspoons plain low-fat or nonfat yogurt
6 sprigs of fresh dill

Preheat the oven to 425°F. Divide the pizza dough into 6 equal pieces. Roll out each piece into a 6- or 7-inch circle and transfer to a baking sheet.

Sprinkle the dough with the cheese. Arrange the onion and tomato slices on top. Bake for 10 to 12 minutes, until the crust is golden. Top each mini pizza with smoked salmon, yogurt, and fresh dill. Serve warm.

YOUTH NUTRIENTS PER SERVING

Calories	387
Calcium	497 mg
Vitamin C	10 mg
Beta-carotene	637 IU

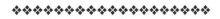

FABULOUS FISH FOR HEALTH

Fish is both high in protein, calcium, and mood-boosting chemicals. But there's more. Fish is also very high in selenium, an antioxidant that protects your cells and chases away the blues. Salmon, tuna, trout, and sardines are good.

SCRAMBLED BURRITOS

Makes 4 servings

Cooking spray
1 onion, chopped fine
2 teaspoons chopped basil
2 teaspoons chopped parsley
1 cup liquid egg substitute
½ cup shredded low-fat or nonfat Cheddar cheese
4 tortillas
4 tablespoons salsa

In a medium skillet sprayed with a little cooking spray, cook the onion over medium heat until soft.

In a small bowl, combine the basil, parsley, onion, egg substitute, and cheese. Pour into the skillet. Cook, stirring lightly, until the egg substitute is set.

Divide evenly among the tortillas. Fold each tortilla over the egg mixture and top with salsa. Serve hot.

YOUTH NUTRIENTS PER SERVING

Calories	222
Calcium	219 mg
Vitamin C	3 mg
Beta-carotene	1,708 IU

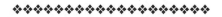

HEALTHY HERBS

Both basil and parsley are loaded with antioxidants, but you need to store them properly so as not to lose their health benefits. Basil can be stored for 5 days in your fridge, wrapped in a damp paper towel and sealed in a plastic vegetable bag. Parsley can be stored for 3 days in your fridge. Put the stems into a glass of cold water.

SOUTH-OF-THE-BORDER SALSA

Makes 6 servings

6 juicy ripe tomatoes, chopped
⅓ cup chopped jalapeño pepper
1 onion, chopped
3 garlic cloves, minced
6 ounces cilantro, chopped
¼ cup chopped parsley

In a large bowl, combine all the ingredients and chill. Serve cold.

YOUTH NUTRIENTS PER SERVING

Calories	35
Calcium	69 mg
Vitamin C	35.5 mg
Beta-carotene	236 IU

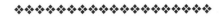

GET YOUR VEGGIE VACCINES AND LIVE LONGER

There's some excitement at Texas A&M University because researchers have developed a vaccine engineered from spuds that can help fight infections. So far only mice have been tested, but human trials may be on the way soon.

IF IT'S GREEN, IT'S GUACAMOLE

Makes 6 servings

1 10-ounce package frozen peas, thawed
1 tomato, chopped fine
4 tablespoons finely chopped onion
3 tablespoons finely chopped cilantro
1 garlic clove, chopped
2 tablespoons plain nonfat yogurt
2 tablespoons lime juice
Dash of hot pepper sauce

Combine all the ingredients in a food processor or blender and process until smooth. Heap into a bowl. Serve at room temperature.

YOUTH NUTRIENTS PER SERVING

Calories	23
Calcium	27 mg
Vitamin C	13 mg
Beta-carotene	216 IU

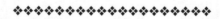

SKINNY SKIN

If you have a history of skin cancer, try reducing your fat to 20 percent of your total diet. In a study it was found that a lower-fat diet reduced the occurrence of precancerous skin lesions.

STUFFED BABY SPUDS

Makes 24 servings

1½ pounds (12) new potatoes, scrubbed
2 tablespoons part skim milk ricotta cheese
2 tablespoons plain low-fat or nonfat yogurt
1 tablespoon chopped dill
½ teaspoon lemon juice
1 tablespoon chopped chives

Cook the new potatoes in their skins. Drain and cut in half. Take a tiny slice off the bottoms so they stand without falling over.

In a small bowl, combine the ricotta cheese, yogurt, dill, lemon juice, and chives. Put a dollop of the mixture on top of each tiny potato half. Serve warm or at room temperature.

YOUTH NUTRIENTS PER SERVING

Calories	25
Calcium	10 mg
Vitamin C	6 mg
Beta-carotene	11 IU

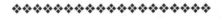

THE "EYES" HAVE IT

A new study from Harvard Medical School found that people who ate foods rich in carotenoids, like sweet potatoes, squash, spinach and other dark leafy green vegetables, had a 43 percent lower risk of macular degeneration, a disease of the aging eye.

BONE BUILDER SPINACH DIP

Makes 24 servings

1 10-ounce package frozen spinach, drained
2 8-ounce containers plain low-fat or nonfat yogurt
1 onion, shredded
¼ cup chopped dill
¼ cup chopped parsley

In a bowl, combine all the ingredients. Mix well. Chill and serve with vegetables or low-fat crackers.

YOUTH NUTRIENTS PER SERVING

Calories	18
Calcium	72 mg
Vitamin C	4 mg
Beta-carotene	1,064 IU

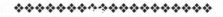

LOW-CAL GREENS

Greens pack a powerful antioxidant punch and go easy on the calories, too. Check these out.

SALAD GREENS	CALORIES PER OUNCE
Asparagus	7
Broccoli	13
Cabbage	5
Celery	2
Cucumber	3
Leeks	6
Lettuce	4

CASBAH DIP

Makes 12 servings

2 19-ounce cans chickpeas, drained
¼ cup lemon juice
4 garlic cloves, peeled
1 tablespoon Dijon mustard
2 tablespoons water

Place all the ingredients in a food processor or blender and process until smooth. Turn out into a bowl and chill. Serve with wedges of pita bread or fresh vegetables.

YOUTH NUTRIENTS PER SERVING

Calories	12
Calcium	3 mg
Vitamin C	1 mg
Beta-carotene	2 IU

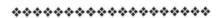

WE'RE SNACKIN' HEALTHIER THESE DAYS

Did you know that pretzel consumption has doubled since 1988? Pretzels are the fastest-growing snack food in the United States.

TROPICAL SALSA

Makes 24 servings

1 mango, peeled and chopped
1 green pepper, seeded and chopped
1 onion, chopped
1 jalapeño pepper, seeded and chopped
1 tablespoon lime juice
1 tablespoon lemon juice

In a bowl, combine all the ingredients. Chill in the fridge before serving.

YOUTH NUTRIENTS PER SERVING

Calories	9
Calcium	4 mg
Vitamin C	10 mg
Beta-carotene	370 IU

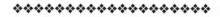

WHERE'S THE HEAT?

Peppers have many antioxidant properties. Here's a wonderful place to find the best and the most: Check out the National Fiery Foods Show in Albuquerque, New Mexico, in March.

SIMPLY SENSATIONAL SALSA

Makes 24 servings

4 tomatoes, chopped fine
4 jalapeño peppers, chopped fine
4 garlic cloves, peeled and chopped fine
2 onions, chopped
2 tablespoons lime juice
2 tablespoons red wine vinegar
1 tablespoon olive oil

Combine all the ingredients in a bowl and chill until ready to serve.

YOUTH NUTRIENTS PER SERVING

Calories	16
Calcium	9 mg
Vitamin C	23 mg
Beta-carotene	186 IU

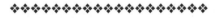

SECONDHAND SMOKERS

Fifteen percent of lung cancer deaths occur in nonsmokers. Yale University School of Medicine researchers found that cancer patients were less likely to eat a diet high in fresh antioxidant-rich vegetables.

SWEET POTATO STICKS

Makes 4 servings

1 teaspoon olive oil
1 teaspoon garlic salt
½ teaspoon paprika
4 sweet potatoes, scrubbed and cut into thin sticks

Preheat the oven to 450°F.

In a large bowl, combine the oil, garlic salt, and paprika. Add the sweet potato sticks and toss until the potatoes are well coated.

Transfer the coated potatoes to a baking sheet and bake 15 minutes. Turn and continue baking for another 15 minutes, or until the potatoes are golden. Place on a serving dish and serve hot.

YOUTH NUTRIENTS PER SERVING

Calories	147
Calcium	29 mg
Vitamin C	30 mg
Beta-carotene	26,256 IU

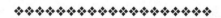

CAN YOU REALLY EAT MORE AND WEIGH LESS?

Yes, say researchers at Vanderbilt University School of Medicine. If you eat low-fat you'll lose about nine pounds in four months. If you eat low-fat <u>and</u> low-cal you'll lose eighteen pounds plus in the same time frame.

BLUSHING SLAW

Makes 6 servings

1 head of red cabbage, shredded
2 bunches of green onions, chopped
1 8-ounce bottle nonfat Italian dressing
1 teaspoon lemon juice
Dash of pepper

In large bowl, combine all the ingredients and chill.

YOUTH NUTRIENTS PER SERVING

Calories	83
Calcium	83 mg
Vitamin C	88 mg
Beta-carotene	86 IU

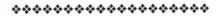

PUT AWAY THOSE MINTS . . . ONION BREATH IS A SIGN OF HEALTH

Researchers at the State University of New York in Albany found that onions reduce the risk of clots that can lead to strokes and heart attacks. Other studies show that people who eat onions regularly have a lower incidence of cancer in the digestive tract.

NO LETTUCE? NO PROBLEM SALAD

Makes 4 servings

18 cherry tomatoes, sliced in half
2 celery stalks, sliced
2 carrots, sliced
1 cucumber, peeled and sliced
1 tablespoon oregano
2 tablespoons red wine vinegar
1 8-ounce bottle nonfat Italian salad dressing
Dash of pepper

Combine all the ingredients in a large salad bowl and toss until the vegetables are well coated. Chill.

YOUTH NUTRIENTS PER SERVING

Calories	169
Calcium	68 mg
Vitamin C	78 mg
Beta-carotene	12,644 IU

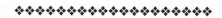

A TOMATO A DAY

New studies show that it may be tomatoes as in tomato sauce served over pasta or sliced up with mozzarella cheese that are the secret to the longer, healthier lives of those who enjoy a Mediterranean diet. Tomatoes have been shown to contain an antioxidant that fights cancer. How many tomatoes offer protection? Researchers figure one a day.

EDITA'S FAVORITE CHEF'S SALAD BOWL

Makes 1 serving

1 cup romaine lettuce, cut into bite-size pieces
1 cup fresh spinach, washed, dried, and cut into bite-size pieces
1 tomato, cut in wedges
½ red pepper, sliced in rings
¼ cup finely chopped parsley
¼ cup finely chopped green onion
1 ounce part skim milk mozzarella cheese, sliced in thin straws
2 ounces skinless turkey light meat, sliced in thin straws

Place all the ingredients in a large salad bowl and toss together. Serve with your favorite nonfat salad dressing on the side.

YOUTH NUTRIENTS PER SERVING

Calories	251
Calcium	338 mg
Vitamin C	146 mg
Beta-carotene	11,885 IU

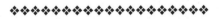

HIS AND HERS VEGGIES

Women need more lettuce, oranges, lemons, grapefruit, squash, and sweet potatoes—loaded with breast cancer fighters. Men need more garlic, onions, brussels sprouts, broccoli, and cauliflower—loaded with colon cancer fighters.

"THINK PICNIC" PASTA SALAD

Makes 4 servings

3 cups cooked pasta elbows or spirals
1 cup broccoli florets
½ cup thinly sliced carrots
½ cup fresh or frozen peas, thawed
½ cup finely chopped parsley
8 ounces plain low-fat yogurt
½ cup grated Parmesan cheese
2 garlic cloves, chopped fine
1 tablespoon Dijon mustard

Put all the ingredients into a large salad bowl and mix until thoroughly blended. Chill. Serve cold.

YOUTH NUTRIENTS PER SERVING

Calories	384
Calcium	276 mg
Vitamin C	45 mg
Beta-carotene	6,323 IU

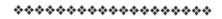

CURIOUS CARROT COMMENTS

Americans consume an average of eight pounds of carrots a year each! One average carrot supplies over 18,000 international units (IU) of beta-carotene. Beta-carotene in carrots has been shown to reduce heart disease and prevent certain forms of blindness.

Here's an interesting bit of carrot trivia: Ever wonder why some carrots in the grocery store are blunt on the bottom? Guess no more. They are grown that way so their pointy little ends don't puncture the plastic bags they are sold in.

FRESH ASPARAGUS SALAD

Makes 4 servings

2 pounds fresh asparagus spears
2 tablespoons nonfat Caesar dressing
1 teaspoon Dijon mustard
2 tablespoons grated Parmesan cheese
Lemon wedges for garnish

Cut off the hard ends of the asparagus stems. Place the asparagus in a steamer basket and steam for 2 to 3 minutes. Make sure the asparagus is still crisp and green. Remove from the steamer and rinse under cold water. Pat dry and arrange on a plate. In a small bowl, mix the dressing and the Dijon mustard together. Pour over the asparagus. Sprinkle the top with the cheese and garnish with lemon wedges.

YOUTH NUTRIENTS PER SERVING

Calories	65
Calcium	83 mg
Vitamin C	30 mg
Beta-carotene	1,341 IU

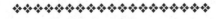

SALAD OF THE GODS

Greeks and Romans believed in the medicinal powers of asparagus and used it in salads and cooking 2,500 years ago. These spears are considered a delicacy and add loads of vitamin C and beta-carotene without adding fat or many calories.

CRIMSON CRUNCH SALAD

Makes 6 servings

3 pints cherry tomatoes, cut in half
1 onion, sliced into very thin rings and separated
½ cup finely chopped fresh basil
¼ cup Bacos®
½ cup low-calorie Italian salad dressing

In a large bowl, combine all the ingredients. Toss well to mix.

YOUTH NUTRIENTS PER SERVING

Calories	89
Calcium	41 mg
Vitamin C	36 mg
Beta-carotene	1,258 IU

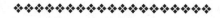

LOW-FAT + VEGETARIAN = HEALTHY HEARTS

A research project at the St. Helena Hospital and Health Center found that a low-fat vegetarian diet plus exercise and weight loss can lower cholesterol and blood pressure in just 12 days!

SKINNY ANTIPASTO SALAD

Makes 4 servings

1 red pepper, cored, seeded, and sliced into thin strips
1 green pepper, cored, seeded, and sliced into thin strips
1 yellow pepper, cored, seeded, and sliced into thin strips
1 garlic clove, minced
¼ cup low-calorie Italian salad dressing

Arrange the peppers in a circular pattern by color on a plate. Sprinkle with the garlic and salad dressing.

YOUTH NUTRIENTS PER SERVING

Calories	39
Calcium	10 mg
Vitamin C	137 mg
Beta-carotene	1,282 IU

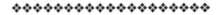

GARLIC FIGHTS STOMACH CANCER BIG TIME

A study by University of Texas cancer researchers at the M. D. Anderson Cancer Center in Houston found that garlic fights the growth of stomach cancer cells.

BERRY SWEET SALAD

Makes 4 servings

1 cantaloupe, peeled, seeded, and cut into chunks
1 honeydew melon, peeled, seeded, and cut into chunks
1 cup blueberries, washed
½ cup raspberries, washed
3 tablespoons raspberry vinegar
2 tablespoons apple juice

In a large glass bowl, combine all the ingredients. Toss well to coat. Chill and toss once more before serving.

YOUTH NUTRIENTS PER SERVING

Calories	193
Calcium	41 mg
Vitamin C	145 mg
Beta-carotene	4,489 IU

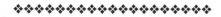

VITAMIN E AND DRINKERS AND SMOKERS

More anti-aging news for vitamin E: Researchers at the University of Arizona feel that vitamin E may protect people who drink alcohol from cancer of the throat, a cancer that is exacerbated by smoking.

FRESHEST, GREENEST GARDEN SALAD

Makes 4 servings

1 cup romaine lettuce leaves, washed and cut into bite-size pieces
1 cup red leaf lettuce, washed and cut into bite-size pieces
1 cup spinach, washed and cut into bite-size pieces
1 cup Boston lettuce, washed and cut into bite-size pieces
¼ cup finely chopped parsley
1 red pepper, washed, seeded, and cut into thin strips
⅓ cup low-calorie Italian salad dressing
¼ cup grated Parmesan cheese

In a large bowl, combine all the ingredients. Toss well to coat.

YOUTH NUTRIENTS PER SERVING

Calories	76
Calcium	176 mg
Vitamin C	52 mg
Beta-carotene	3,677 IU

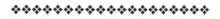

GREAT SALAD MUNCHIES

Pita chips: Take 3 pita breads. Separate each into 2 rounds. Cut each round into 8 pieces. Place them in a single layer on a cookie sheet. Brush with a mixture of lemon juice and crushed garlic. Spray lightly with cooking spray. Bake at 350°F. for 15 minutes, or until lightly browned. Munch a bunch with your favorite salad.

SWEET POTATO SALAD

Makes 4 servings

2 sweet potatoes, cooked, peeled, and sliced like French fries
¼ cup raisins
1 tablespoon lemon juice
1 garlic clove, chopped fine
2 teaspoons honey
¼ teaspoon cinnamon
¼ teaspoon ground ginger
¼ cup finely chopped parsley

Place the sliced potatoes in a shallow dish. Combine the remaining ingredients and pour over the potatoes. Serve at once.

YOUTH NUTRIENTS PER SERVING

Calories	121
Calcium	78 mg
Vitamin C	22 mg
Beta-carotene	13,918 IU

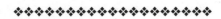

FLYING MAKING YOU SICK?

A recent study of airsickness found that eating low-calorie, low-fat foods like breads and cereals can cut down on the queasies in the air. So give a pass to the salty snacks and bring out your own bagel.

MEDITERRANEAN TUNA SALAD

Makes 4 servings

¼ cup low-calorie Italian salad dressing
4 tablespoons grated Parmesan cheese
8 cups romaine lettuce, cut into chunks
1 6⅛-ounce can tuna packed in water, drained
1 onion, sliced
3 tomatoes, cut into chunks
4 black olives, halved

In a large bowl, mix the salad dressing and cheese together. Add the rest of the ingredients and toss well to coat. Serve.

YOUTH NUTRIENTS PER SERVING

Calories	123
Calcium	94 mg
Vitamin C	46 mg
Beta-carotene	3,576 IU

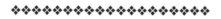

KISS AND LOSE WEIGHT

Did you know that the average kiss burns between 6 and 12 calories? Go ahead, pucker up!

CRUNCHY SPINACH SALAD

Makes 4 servings

2 cups romaine lettuce, washed and torn into bite-size pieces
2 cups spinach, washed and torn into bite-size pieces
8 cherry tomatoes, washed and halved
2 apples, peeled and chopped fine
1 onion, chopped fine
2 tablespoons cider vinegar
2 tablespoons olive oil

Combine all the ingredients in a large bowl. Toss well to coat. Serve.

YOUTH NUTRIENTS PER SERVING

Calories	195
Calcium	78 mg
Vitamin C	89 mg
Beta-carotene	4,896 IU

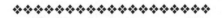

BETA-CAROTENE IS BETTER IN FOOD

THAN IN SUPPLEMENTS, SAY EXPERTS

Some good choices:

Tomato juice
Spinach
Sweet potatoes
Watermelon
Carrots
Pumpkin

SPUD SOUP

Makes 6 servings

1 can chicken broth
1 can cream of potato soup
1 carrot, peeled and sliced in thin rounds
1 cup broccoli florets
1 can evaporated skim milk
6 ounces low-fat Cheddar cheese

Combine the chicken broth, cream of potato soup, carrot, and broccoli in a medium saucepan and simmer until the vegetables are tender, about 3 to 5 minutes. Reduce the heat and add the evaporated skim milk and cheese. Mix through and heat, but do not boil. Serve when the cheese has just melted.

YOUTH NUTRIENTS PER SERVING

Calories	136
Calcium	288 mg
Vitamin C	19 mg
Beta-carotene	4,326 IU

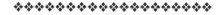

CHEESE TIDBITS

According to the University of California at Berkeley's <u>Wellness Letter,</u> "Americans eat more than twice as much cheese today as in the late 1960s— 28 pounds per capita each year. One survey found that people cutting back on fat find cheese the most difficult food to trim from their diets. And thanks to the national fondness for pizza, mozzarella is now the second most popular cheese in the U.S. after cheddar."

NEW YORK'S FINEST SOUP

Makes 4 servings

4 cups chicken broth
½ pound smoked salmon, chopped into bits
½ cup chopped green onion
½ cup fresh spinach, rinsed, drained, and chopped into bits
¼ cup chopped fresh dill
Dash of pepper

In a medium saucepan, combine the broth, salmon, and green onion. Bring to a boil, cover, and simmer for 10 minutes. Add the spinach, dill, and pepper. Simmer another 2 to 3 minutes. Serve hot.

YOUTH NUTRIENTS PER SERVING

Calories	157
Calcium	92 mg
Vitamin C	4 mg
Beta-carotene	568 IU

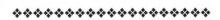

WINNING THE VEGETABLE HATERS WARS

If your family finds vegetables a turnoff try these tricks to make them more appealing:

- Simmer vegetables in a little chicken broth instead of water.
- Cook vegetables in a little orange or apple juice to sweeten them up and change the flavor a little.
- Throw vegetables into tomato sauce. They will improve the nutritional value of the sauce and the rich tomato flavor will mask the strong flavor of many vegetables.

HALLOWEEN SOUP

Makes 6 servings

1 medium butternut squash, peeled, seeded, and cut into chunks
1 onion, chopped
1 apple, peeled, cored, and cut into chunks
2 16-ounce cans chicken broth
1 bay leaf
1 teaspoon thyme
¼ cup orange juice
¼ cup lemon juice
Dash of pepper to taste

Place all the ingredients in a large saucepan. Simmer for 30 minutes, until the squash and apple are soft. Remove the bay leaf and transfer the soup to a blender or food processor and process until smooth. Pour into bowls and serve hot.

YOUTH NUTRIENTS PER SERVING

Calories	78
Calcium	76 mg
Vitamin C	36 mg
Beta-carotene	8,908 IU

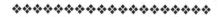

FRIGHT NIGHT FOR CANCER CELLS

Scientists at the Hollings Cancer Center at the Medical University of South Carolina found that beta-carotene in broccoli, carrots, spinach, squash, and sweet potatoes seems to interrupt and reverse the out-of-control cell pattern that changes the cycle of normal cells into the destructive pattern of cancer cells.

SOUTH-OF-THE-BORDER CHICKEN SOUP

Makes 4 servings

1 package dry chicken noodle soup mix
½ cup salsa
4 tablespoons shredded low-fat Cheddar cheese
4 teaspoons finely chopped green pepper

In a medium saucepan, heat 3½ cups of water to boiling. Stir in the chicken soup mix and salsa and reduce the heat to low. Cover and simmer for 8 minutes, or until the noodles are soft. Pour into 4 bowls and top each serving with the Cheddar cheese and green pepper.

Youth Nutrients Per Serving

Calories	97
Calcium	94 mg
Vitamin C	4 mg
Beta-carotene	313 IU

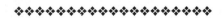

EATING OUT CAN BE GOOD FOR YOU

Fast Food: Grilled chicken sandwich
Chinese: Wonton soup, stir-fried vegetables
Italian: Pasta with red or white clam sauce
Sandwiches: Turkey on rye, hold the mayo
Mexican: Chicken fajitas

FOUNTAIN OF YOUTH VEGGIE BROTH

Makes 8 servings

2 leeks, washed and sliced thin
1 onion, peeled and sliced
4 carrots, peeled and sliced
4 garlic cloves, peeled and mashed
1 bunch of parsley, washed
2 celery stalks, washed and chopped
½ head of cabbage, sliced
1 sweet potato, peeled and sliced
½ teaspoon thyme
½ teaspoon oregano
2 bay leaves
1 teaspoon peppercorns

Place all the ingredients in a large kettle with 9 cups of cold water and bring to a boil. Turn down the heat and simmer for 1 hour, or until all the vegetables are soft. Strain through a strainer.

YOUTH NUTRIENTS PER SERVING

Calories	95
Calcium	196 mg
Vitamin C	51 mg
Beta-carotene	15,289 IU

❖❖❖❖❖❖❖❖❖❖❖❖❖❖❖❖❖❖❖

AMERICANS' MOST HATED VEGETABLES

Brussels sprouts
Spinach
Asparagus
Broccoli
Cauliflower

GLORIOUS GAZPACHO

Makes 4 servings

3 cups tomato juice
1 cup vegetable juice cocktail
4 garlic cloves, peeled and chopped fine
¼ cup finely chopped parsley
Dash of Tabasco sauce
2 yellow peppers, seeded and chopped fine
2 cucumbers, peeled, seeded, and chopped fine
2 celery stalks, chopped fine
4 tomatoes, chopped coarsely

In a large bowl, combine all the ingredients. Stir and chill until ready to serve.

YOUTH NUTRIENTS PER SERVING

Calories	133
Calcium	133 mg
Vitamin C	260 mg
Beta-carotene	3,952 IU

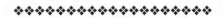

ANOTHER FASCINATING FACT

Tortillas are now the fastest-growing segment of the baking industry. We all munched about 60 billion tortillas in 1995 and that isn't even counting tortilla chips. That's 225 tortillas per person—more than bagels, English muffins, and pitas combined. Some of us had more than our share, right?

CELADON SOUP

Makes 4 servings

1 can (8 ounces) chicken broth
1 celery stalk, chopped fine
1 onion, chopped fine
1 carrot, peeled and chopped fine
2 cups broccoli florets
2 cups skinless, boneless chicken breast pieces
1 can cream of potato soup

In a medium saucepan over medium-high heat, place the chicken stock, water, celery, onion, carrot, broccoli, and chicken. Bring to a boil. Turn down the heat, cover, and simmer for about 10 minutes, until the vegetables are tender. Turn down the heat again and stir in the cream of potato soup. Serve at once.

YOUTH NUTRIENTS PER SERVING

Calories	206
Calcium	72 mg
Vitamin C	47 mg
Beta-carotene	6,423 IU

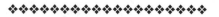

GET A HANDLE ON A SERVING

√ I cup raw leafy vegetables
√ ½ cup cooked vegetables
√ I medium potato
√ I carrot
√ I apple, banana, pear, orange
√ 3 apricots
√ ½ grapefruit
√ ½ cup cantaloupe

PIZZA SOUP

Makes 8 servings

2 onions, chopped fine
1 green pepper, seeded and chopped fine
1 red pepper, seeded and chopped fine
1 can (8 ounces) beef broth
1 16-ounce can tomatoes
4 ounces pizza sauce
1 cup sliced mushrooms
1 teaspoon Italian seasoning
½ cup part skim milk shredded mozzarella cheese

Combine all the ingredients except the cheese in a medium saucepan and bring to a boil. Cover and simmer for 15 minutes, until all the vegetables are tender. Pour into bowls, top with the cheese, and serve.

YOUTH NUTRIENTS PER SERVING

Calories	67
Calcium	90 mg
Vitamin C	38 mg
Beta-carotene	1,109 IU

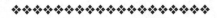

EATING WITH FRIENDS MAY BE DANGEROUS TO YOUR DIET

A new study from the University of Toronto found that women who ate alone averaged about 375 calories. When they ate with friends they averaged 700 calories. Most of the extra calories came from dessert. Surprised? I wasn't either.

VEGGIES WITH ATTITUDE

Serves 6

2 16-ounce packages frozen mixed vegetables
¼ cup boiling water
⅓ cup low-fat Italian salad dressing
Dash of hot sauce

In a heavy skillet, cook the vegetables in the boiling water until they are tender but still crisp, about 15 minutes. Drain. Return the vegetables to the pot. Pour the salad dressing and a dash of hot sauce over the vegetables and toss to coat. Cook for a minute until the vegetables are heated through.

YOUTH NUTRIENTS PER SERVING

Calories	111
Calcium	38 mg
Vitamin C	16 mg
Beta-carotene	7,678 IU

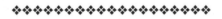

GIVE YOURSELF AN ANTI-AGING BREAK

Plan ahead. Chop up lots of peppers, carrots, broccoli, and cantaloupe and have it ready in the fridge for when you get a snack attack. That way you won't reach for junk food, you'll reach for "youth food."

CHEDDAR MASHED SPUDS

Serves 8

8 baking potatoes
2 cups low-fat shredded Cheddar cheese
¼ cup liquid Butter Buds®
4 ounces plain nonfat yogurt
4 ounces nonfat sour cream
2 tablespoons chopped green onion
Dash of pepper
Cooking spray

Preheat the oven to 325°F. In a large Dutch oven, bring the potatoes to a boil. Turn down the heat and simmer, covered, until almost tender. Drain, peel, and grate. In a large bowl, combine the potatoes, cheese, Butter Buds®, yogurt, sour cream, green onions, and pepper. Transfer the mixture to a 2-quart nonstick casserole sprayed with cooking spray and bake for 45 minutes. Serve hot.

YOUTH NUTRIENTS PER SERVING

Calories	217
Calcium	238 mg
Vitamin C	30 mg
Beta-carotene	78 IU

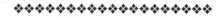

"I'VE GOT GOOD NEWS . . . AND BAD NEWS"

First the good news: According to statistics, we are eating more low-fat foods, such as pasta and fruit, and less fat food, such as hot dogs. Now the bad news: We are all ten pounds heavier than we were ten years ago. Go figure. Could it be the couch potato syndrome? Could it be more calories? Yes to both!

HERBED TOMATO GLOBES

Serves 4

Cooking spray
2 large tomatoes, sliced in half
1 teaspoon olive oil
2 tablespoons chopped parsley
½ teaspoon oregano
½ teaspoon basil
4 teaspoons grated Parmesan cheese

Preheat the oven to 350°F. Spray a 9 x 9-inch baking pan with cooking spray. Place the tomatoes, cut side up, on the pan. Drizzle with olive oil and sprinkle with the spices. Bake for 20 minutes. After 20 minutes, turn on the broiler and sprinkle the tomatoes with the Parmesan cheese. Broil until the cheese turns golden. Serve hot.

YOUTH NUTRIENTS PER SERVING

Calories	37
Calcium	60 mg
Vitamin C	14 mg
Beta-carotene	863 IU

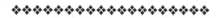

TOMATOES VS. PROSTATE CANCER

A recent study shows that men who ate at least five tomatoes a week had a 40 percent lower risk of developing prostate cancer. The secret is a substance in tomatoes that may be a twin to beta-carotene, the cancer fighter found in carrots.

SPICY SWEET POTATO CAKES

Serves 6

2 sweet potatoes, cooked, peeled, and cut into chunks
1 tablespoon grated fresh ginger
1 tablespoon curry powder
1 teaspoon low-sodium soy sauce
1 tablespoon finely chopped garlic
½ cup skim milk
Cooking spray

Place all the ingredients except the cooking spray into the bowl of a food processor or blender and process until smooth. Form into patties. Fry on a skillet lightly coated with cooking spray until crisp. Turn and cook until the other side is crisp. Serve hot.

YOUTH NUTRIENTS PER SERVING

Calories	57
Calcium	36 mg
Vitamin C	10 mg
Beta-carotene	8,737 IU

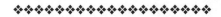

ANTI-AGING CRAVINGS

Studies show that women crave sweet, high-fat foods when the winter blues hit, while men go for more savory snacks. The cravings are linked to the production of melatonin, a mood-elevating and youth-enhancing hormone produced in the brain.

HONG KONG SWEET POTATOES

Makes 8 servings

8 medium sweet potatoes
1 tablespoon grated fresh ginger
1 garlic clove
Dash of low-sodium soy sauce
Dash of pepper
¼ cup chicken broth

Place the potatoes in a large saucepan, cover with water, and cook until tender for about 20 minutes. Drain, peel, and mash. Keep the potatoes warm.

In a small saucepan, cook the ginger, garlic, soy sauce, and pepper in the chicken broth until soft.

Pour the ginger mixture into the mashed potatoes and mix well. Serve at once.

Youth Nutrients Per Serving

Calories	140
Calcium	30 mg
Vitamin C	30 mg
Beta-carotene	26,082 IU

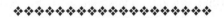

THE LOWDOWN ON SWEET POTATOES

If you thought sweet potatoes were loaded with fat and sugar because of their name you would be wrong. On the contrary. Sweet potatoes only sound fattening. Here are the facts:

- Sweet potatoes contain the same number of calories as white potatoes—130 calories per 4 ounces.
- They contain 50 percent of the RDA for vitamin C.
- They contain three times the RDA for beta-carotene.
- They are virtually fat-free.
- Here's a bonus: They have more potassium than a banana.

BUBBLE AND SQUEAK

Makes 4 servings

1 pound potatoes, peeled and cut into chunks
1 onion, chopped
Cooking spray
¾ cup skim milk
3 cups warm cabbage, cooked and chopped fine

Boil the potatoes in a medium pot in a little salted water. While the potatoes are cooking, sauté the onion until golden in a small skillet that has
been sprayed with the cooking spray. When the potatoes are soft, drain
them and return them to the pot with the skim milk. Mash the potatoes.
Stir in the onion and cabbage. Serve warm.

YOUTH NUTRIENTS PER SERVING

Calories	125
Calcium	106 mg
Vitamin C	51 mg
Beta-carotene	160 IU

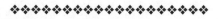

GETTING OLDER YOUNGER

Over 25 percent of our kids don't eat veggies on any given day. So what? So
these kids are not getting the benefits of life-extending antioxidants and are
getting older younger.

SUPER SUPPER SPUDS

Makes 4 servings

2 baking potatoes, baked
2 cups broccoli florets, steamed
½ cup part skim ricotta cheese
2 tablespoons shredded low-fat or nonfat Cheddar cheese
½ cup salsa

Preheat the oven to 375°F.

Cut the baked potatoes in half and scoop out the insides. In a large bowl, combine the hot potatoes, steamed broccoli, ricotta cheese, Cheddar cheese, and salsa. Mix to combine. Fill the potato shells with the mixture. On a cookie sheet or piece of foil, place the potatoes in the oven. Bake for 20 to 30 minutes, until hot through and through. Serve.

YOUTH NUTRIENTS PER SERVING

Calories	147
Calcium	147 mg
Vitamin C	69 mg
Beta-carotene	1,455 IU

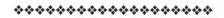

WOMEN AGAINST MEAT

American women are eliminating meat from our diets faster than men. Way to go, ladies!

TOMATO PUDDING

Makes 8 servings

2 28-ounce cans seasoned tomatoes
8 slices day-old white bread, cut into cubes

Preheat the oven to 375°F.

In an 8-inch square baking dish, place half of the tomatoes. On top, place half of the bread cubes. Repeat. The final layer should be bread cubes. Bake for 30 minutes, until the tomatoes are bubbling and the top is golden.

YOUTH NUTRIENTS PER SERVING

Calories	106
Calcium	79 mg
Vitamin C	30 mg
Beta-carotene	1,199 IU

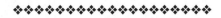

FAT IS GAINING ON US

A new Harris Poll shows that a record 71 percent of us aged twenty-five and older are overweight today, compared with 69 percent in 1994 and 56 percent in 1984.

ROMAN BROCCOLI

Makes 4 servings

4 garlic cloves, chopped fine
¼ cup chicken broth
2 bunches of broccoli, chopped
1 red pepper, seeded and sliced into slivers
¼ cup finely chopped parsley
1 tablespoon grated Parmesan cheese

In a skillet over medium heat, sauté the garlic in a little of the chicken broth until golden. Add a little more chicken broth and the broccoli. Continue cooking for about 5 minutes, until the broccoli is tender-crisp. Add the rest of the chicken broth and the red pepper. Cook for another 2 minutes. Sprinkle the parsley and the Parmesan cheese on top, toss, and serve.

YOUTH NUTRIENTS PER SERVING

Calories	43
Calcium	101 mg
Vitamin C	82 mg
Beta-carotene	2,617 IU

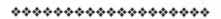

STEAMED VEGGIES TIMETABLE

Broccoli takes 10 to 15 minutes.
Carrots take 10 to 15 minutes.
Spinach takes 3 minutes.
Cauliflower takes 10 to 15 minutes.

GARLICKY COLLARD GREENS

Makes 2 servings

1 pound collard greens, washed and chopped
4 garlic cloves, chopped
1 onion, chopped
Cooking spray

In a large pot with a steamer, steam the collard greens for 5 to 7 minutes, until tender. While the greens are steaming, sauté the garlic and onion until golden in a small skillet sprayed with the cooking spray. Place the collard greens in a serving bowl, pour the onion and garlic on top, and toss to mix well. Serve hot.

YOUTH NUTRIENTS PER SERVING

Calories	93
Calcium	115 mg
Vitamin C	58 mg
Beta-carotene	7,559 IU

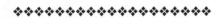

SAFE STORAGE

- Fresh eggs keep in the fridge for 3 to 5 weeks.
- Mayo salads keep in the fridge for 3 to 5 days.
- Opened lunch meats keep in the fridge for 3 to 5 days.
- Uncooked meat keeps in the fridge for 3 to 5 days.
- Ground meat keeps in the fridge for 1 to 2 days.
- Milk keeps in the fridge for 5 days after the expiration date.

NO FUSS GRILLED OR BROILED VEGGIES

Makes 4 servings

1 red pepper, seeded and cut into chunks
1 green pepper, seeded and cut into chunks
1 yellow pepper, seeded and cut into chunks
1 red onion, peeled and cut into chunks
1 eggplant (about 12 ounces), cut into slices
1 teaspoon olive oil

Preheat the broiler.

Arrange the veggies on a large sheet of aluminum foil. Drizzle with the olive oil. Fold up the foil, making a sealed package for the veggies. Place on an oven rack about 6 inches from the broiler and cook for 15 minutes. Open carefully and serve.

YOUTH NUTRIENTS PER SERVING

Calories	70
Calcium	22 mg
Vitamin C	141 mg
Beta-carotene	1,354 IU

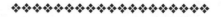

WHY ARE WE FATTER?

Could be that we are scarfing down 14 million burgers, 19 million servings of fries, and 29 million servings of soft drinks in fast-food restaurants. All of this up, way up, from just a few years ago.

GREEN AND ORANGE MIX

Makes 6 servings

3 sweet potatoes, peeled and cut into chunks
½ cup apple juice
1 apple, peeled, seeded, and chopped fine
¼ cup light brown sugar
Dash of Worcestershire sauce
6 ounces spinach, washed and chopped

In medium saucepan, cook the potatoes until tender, about 30 minutes. Drain. Put the potatoes in a large bowl and mash. Set aside and keep warm. In the same pot as you cooked the potatoes, put the apple juice, chopped apple, brown sugar, and Worcestershire sauce. Bring to a boil. Add the spinach. Turn down the heat and simmer for a minute, until the spinach is wilted. Stir the spinach mixture into the mashed potatoes and mix well. Serve hot.

YOUTH NUTRIENTS PER SERVING

Calories	120
Calcium	51 mg
Vitamin C	24 mg
Beta-carotene	14,957 IU

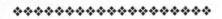

CANCER OF THE MOUTH FOILED

New studies from the former Soviet Union found that beta-carotene can reduce lesions that are part of the symptoms of cancer of the mouth.

ROOTIN' FOR VEGGIES

Makes 8 servings

1 pound potatoes, peeled and cut into chunks
1 sweet potato, peeled and cut into chunks
1 Spanish onion, peeled and cut into chunks
4 carrots, peeled and cut into medium slices
½ pound fresh beets, peeled and cut into chunks
Cooking spray
½ cup chopped parsley

Preheat the oven to 400°F.

In a roasting pan, arrange the vegetables in one layer. Spray lightly with the cooking spray. Toss and spray again. Bake for 45 minutes, turning several times, until tender. Serve hot, sprinkled with parsley.

Youth Nutrients Per Serving

Calories	109
Calcium	82 mg
Vitamin C	26 mg
Beta-carotene	15,398 IU

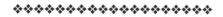

FANCY IT UP WITH STYLE

<u>Green onion fans:</u> Trim off both ends of a green onion. Using a sharp paring knife, make thin slits from the center of the onion out. Drop it into a bowl of ice water until it curls.

<u>Vegetable bowls:</u> Scoop out the insides of peppers, thick cucumber boats, or thick slices of zucchini. Fill with cooked vegetables.

<u>Green cutouts:</u> Cut green pepper into fancy shapes with a cookie cutter.

BAKED CABBAGE

Makes 4 servings

Cooking spray
4 cups shredded cabbage
1 cup peeled and shredded carrot
4 green onions, sliced fine
1 cup skim milk
1 ounce low-fat shredded Cheddar cheese
½ cup liquid egg substitute
¼ cup chopped parsley
2 tablespoons grated Parmesan cheese

Preheat the oven to 375°F.

Spray a small saucepan with the vegetable cooking spray and heat over medium-high heat. Add the cabbage, carrot, and green onions and sauté until crisp, about 5 minutes. Put the cooked vegetables into a casserole or baking dish. In a small bowl, mix together the skim milk, Cheddar cheese, and egg and pour over the vegetables. Sprinkle the top with the parsley and Parmesan cheese. Bake for 45 minutes, or until a knife inserted in the center comes out clean. Serve hot.

YOUTH NUTRIENTS PER SERVING

Calories	179
Calcium	389
Vitamin C	75 mg
Beta-carotene	19,019 IU

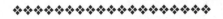

HEARTBURN SOLUTIONS

Fifty-seven percent of married folks suffer from heartburn vs. 13 percent of divorced folks. If you are plagued and don't want to be single, try chewing a sugarless gum. Researchers at the University of Alabama found that chewing sugarless gum after meals stimulates the production of saliva and helps clear away gastric acids that cause heartburn.

BARNYARD STEW

Serves 8

1 pound skinless chicken breasts
1 pound skinless turkey breasts
1 can low-sodium chicken broth
1 can cream of mushroom soup
2 cups sliced carrots
1 cup sliced celery
2 cups frozen peas
2 potatoes, peeled and cut in chunks
2 onions, peeled and cut in chunks
¼ cup chopped parsley
Dash of pepper

Preheat the oven to 375°F.

In a heavy ovenproof casserole, combine all the ingredients. Cover and bake for 1 to 1½ hours, until the stew bubbles and the vegetables are tender. Serve hot.

YOUTH NUTRIENTS PER SERVING

Calories	219
Calcium	62 mg
Vitamin C	26 mg
Beta-carotene	8,054 IU

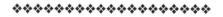

WALK WHILE DINNER COOKS

Can't find time to walk? Pop this recipe in the oven and get moving. You'll lose years and pounds while dinner bakes itself.

- Put on comfortable walking shoes and absorbent socks.
- Maintain a natural pace.
- Bend your elbows and swing your arms a little to get more power.
- Focus on faster steps; your stride will develop naturally.

CLASSIC VEGGIE CHILI

Makes 8 servings

1 onion, chopped
1 red pepper, chopped
1 green pepper, chopped
1 celery stalk, chopped
3 garlic cloves, chopped
¼ cup chicken broth
1 can (30-ounces) tomatoes
2 tablespoons chili powder
Dash of hot pepper sauce to taste
2 15-ounce cans pinto beans, drained

In a large saucepan or Dutch oven, cook the onion, red and green peppers, celery, and garlic in the chicken broth until tender. Add the tomatoes, spices, and pinto beans, cover, and simmer for 5 minutes. Pour into bowls.

YOUTH NUTRIENTS PER SERVING

Calories	123
Calcium	87 mg
Vitamin C	45 mg
Beta-carotene	1,890 IU

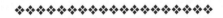

SOME LIKE IT HOT, HOTTER, HOTTEST

The mildest hot peppers are Anaheim.

The hottest hot peppers are habanero.

But there are lots of choices in between like jalapeño, cayenne, and serrano.

P.S. Some studies are finding that hot peppers are good cancer fighters, so stoke up.

SPAGHETTI SQUASH PRIMAVERA

Makes 4 servings

1 medium spaghetti squash
1 tablespoon olive oil
1 onion, chopped
1 red pepper, chopped
1 green pepper, chopped
1 16-ounce can spaghetti sauce
1 16-ounce can seasoned tomatoes
4 garlic cloves, minced
1 cup sliced carrots
2 cups broccoli florets
1 zucchini, sliced
¼ cup ketchup
Dash of pepper
½ cup grated Parmesan cheese
¼ cup chopped parsley

Preheat the oven to 350°F.

Put the squash in a baking dish with a little bit of water to prevent the squash from sticking, pierce the squash with a fork, and bake it for an hour.

When the squash has been in the oven for about 45 minutes, start the primavera sauce. In a large saucepan, heat the oil. Add the chopped onion and cook until the onion is soft. Add the rest of the ingredients except for the Parmesan cheese and parsley. Cover and simmer for 10 minutes.

Take the squash out of the oven, cut it in half lengthwise, and with a fork, scoop out the strands onto a platter. Top the squash with the primavera sauce and toss. Sprinkle the Parmesan cheese and parsley on top. Serve hot.

YOUTH NUTRIENTS PER SERVING

Calories	227
Calcium	316 mg
Vitamin C	152 mg
Beta-carotene	13,084 IU

RAINBOW POTATO DINNER

Makes 4 servings

4 baking potatoes, baked and split in half
1 onion, chopped
1 red pepper, seeded and chopped
1 green pepper, seeded and chopped
¼ cup chicken broth
½ pound ground turkey
1 15-ounce can tomato sauce
¼ cup barbecue sauce
1 15-ounce can corn kernels, drained

While the potatoes are baking, make this topping: In a skillet, cook the onion and red and green peppers in the chicken broth for a couple of minutes, until the onion is transparent. Add the ground turkey and cook until the meat is browned all over. Mix in the tomato sauce, barbecue sauce, and corn. Reduce the heat, cover, and simmer for 5 minutes.

Split the baked potatoes and spoon the topping evenly over the top of each one. Any extra can be served on the side.

YOUTH NUTRIENTS PER SERVING

Calories	260
Calcium	49 mg
Vitamin C	56 mg
Beta-carotene	477 IU

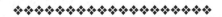

VITAMIN C: THE BODYBUILDER'S VITAMIN

If you are trying to build muscle and lose fat, studies show you need lots of vitamin C. It helps you maintain stamina and youthful body contouring.

NEPTUNE BURGERS

Makes 4 servings

2 14½-ounce cans salmon, drained and flaked
½ cup liquid egg substitute
1¼ cups seasoned bread crumbs
½ cup chopped green onion
1 tablespoon lemon juice
Cooking spray

In a large bowl, combine the salmon, egg substitute, bread crumbs, green onion, and lemon juice. Mix well. Shape into 8 patties. Spray a skillet with cooking spray and fry the patties on both sides, about 3 minutes on each side, until brown. Drain on paper towels.

YOUTH NUTRIENTS PER SERVING

Calories	464
Calcium	516 mg
Vitamin C	4 mg
Beta-carotene	849 IU

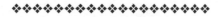

THE GREEN MACHINE

Green onions, scallions, and chives all make a healthy change from regular onions. Powerful anti-aging foods loaded with antioxidants, these little green miracles can really enhance the flavor and goodness of some of your favorite dishes.

- Add some chopped chives, green onions, or scallions to plain nonfat yogurt and use as a baked potato topper.
- Mix some chopped chives, green onions, or scallions into a tub of nonfat cream cheese and use as a spread or dip.

LET'S BE GOOD TONITE VEGGIE PLATTER

Makes 4 servings

4 cups cooked rice
2 cups thinly sliced carrots
1 cup thinly sliced zucchini
2 cups pea pods
½ cup grated Parmesan cheese
1 teaspoon basil

While the rice is cooking according to package directions, prepare the vegetables. In a steamer, steam the carrots for 3 minutes. Add the zucchini and steam for another 3 minutes, then add the pea pods and steam for another 2 minutes. Spoon the rice onto a platter, top with the steamed vegetables, sprinkle with the Parmesan cheese and basil before serving.

YOUTH NUTRIENTS PER SERVING

Calories	372
Calcium	235 mg
Vitamin C	52 mg
Beta-carotene	15,970 IU

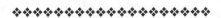

THE GENETIC CONNECTION

If your Mom hated broccoli, chances are you hate it too, and so will your kids and grandkids. Why? New research from the University of Cincinnati finds that genetic factors may influence whether or not we like foods such as broccoli, orange juice, cottage cheese, chicken, and hamburger. But researchers say that when it comes to broccoli, we can all develop a taste for it, no matter what our genes say.

CHICKEN AND VEGGIE WRAPS

Makes 4 servings

3 tablespoons hoisin sauce
2 tablespoons ground ginger
2 garlic cloves, chopped fine
1 pound skinless, boneless chicken breasts, cut into 4 pieces
1 red pepper, seeded and slivered
4 carrots, peeled and sliced thin
1 onion, sliced into thin rings and separated
4 green onions, sliced thick
1 yellow pepper, seeded and slivered
4 cups rice, cooked and kept hot

Preheat the oven to 425°F.

In a small bowl, combine the hoisin sauce, ginger, and garlic. Next, tear off 4 large pieces of aluminum foil. Place a piece of chicken in the center of each and ¼ of the vegetables on top. Drizzle the hoisin sauce mixture over each packet. Seal the packets, place on a large cookie sheet in the oven and bake for 30 minutes. Open carefully and serve with the hot rice.

YOUTH NUTRIENTS PER SERVING

Calories	532
Calcium	194 mg
Vitamin C	163 mg
Beta-carotene	24,289 IU

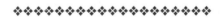

SAY GOOD-BYE TO DRY CHICKEN

Here's a great tip: You know that when you strip the skin off chicken you get rid of a lot of fat. So what's the problem? The problem is dried-out chicken. Not anymore. Just mix up some of your favorite chicken spices with a little plain nonfat or low-fat yogurt and slather on the stripped chicken. Say hello to flavor and good-bye to dry!

SALAD NIÇOISE

Makes 4 servings

¼ cup chopped parsley
¼ cup olive oil
2 tablespoons balsamic vinegar
½ teaspoon Dijon mustard
1 head of romaine lettuce, torn into pieces
½ pound green beans, frozen and thawed and lightly steamed
2 potatoes, cooked and cubed
4 green onions, sliced thin
12 ounces canned tuna, packed in water, drained
1 egg, hard-boiled and quartered
2 tomatoes, cut into 8 wedges
4 olives, halved

In a small bowl, combine the parsley, olive oil, balsamic vinegar, and mustard. Mix to combine and set aside.

Divide the romaine lettuce into 4 portions and place on 4 large dinner plates. Top each plate of lettuce with ¼ of the remaining ingredients. Drizzle the dressing over each and serve.

YOUTH NUTRIENTS PER SERVING

Calories	399
Calcium	263 mg
Vitamin C	95 mg
Beta-carotene	5,761 IU

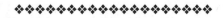

Get those "F Words" Out of Your Vocabulary: fat food, fried food, fast food.
—FLORENCE GRIFFITH JOYNER

CHICKEN FAJITAS

Makes 4 servings

2 skinless, boneless chicken breasts, cut into slices
2 onions, sliced
¼ cup low-calorie Italian salad dressing
4 6-inch tortillas, warmed in the oven
1 cup shredded lettuce
1 cup chopped tomatoes
½ cup shredded low-fat or nonfat mozzarella cheese
½ cup chopped onion
1 cup salsa

In a medium skillet, cook the chicken and sliced onions in the Italian salad dressing until the chicken is cooked, about 5 minutes. Don't forget to keep stirring. Divide the chicken and onion mixture among the 4 tortillas. Fold each tortilla over and serve with the shredded lettuce, chopped tomatoes, mozzarella, chopped onion, and salsa.

YOUTH NUTRIENTS PER SERVING

Calories	321
Calcium	215 mg
Vitamin C	19 mg
Beta-carotene	1,073 IU

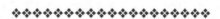

WE'RE TALKING A HEALTH GAME, BUT WE'RE NOT PLAYING

USA Today reports that there is a shrinking niche for lean fast food. Fat fast food is winning.

PRETTY AS A PICTURE CHICKEN KEBABS

Makes 4 servings

24 cherry tomatoes
2 skinless, boneless chicken breasts, cut into bite-size pieces
1 yellow squash, cut into bite-size pieces
16 pearl onions, peeled
8 broccoli florets
4 teaspoons low-calorie Italian salad dressing

Preheat the broiler.

On 8 skewers alternate the tomatoes, chicken, squash, onion, and broccoli. Drizzle with the salad dressing. Broil 20 minutes, turning often, until the chicken is done.

YOUTH NUTRIENTS PER SERVING

Calories	516
Calcium	288 mg
Vitamin C	442 mg
Beta-carotene	11,245 IU

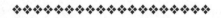

GO EXOTIC

Looking for a change? Looking for a treat? America is eating exotic. Try venison, ostrich, rattlesnake, kangaroo, alligator, and buffalo.

SPICY TURKEY BURGERS

Makes 6 servings

1 pound ground turkey
1 cup salsa
1 cup fresh bread crumbs
1 tablespoon finely chopped cilantro
6 hamburger buns, split and toasted
1 cup shredded lettuce
2 tomatoes, sliced thick
1 onion, sliced thick

In a large bowl, combine the turkey, salsa, bread crumbs, and cilantro. Mix well and shape into 6 patties. Broil the patties under a broiler for 6 minutes per side, or until the center is no longer pink. Place each patty on half a bun and top with lettuce, a tomato slice, and an onion slice. Top with the top half of the bun.

YOUTH NUTRIENTS PER SERVING

Calories	280
Calcium	97 mg
Vitamin C	14 mg
Beta-carotene	712 IU

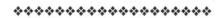

NO, YOU AREN'T HUNGRY

- Drink a big glass of water before each meal.
- Eat very, very, slowly—you won't be hungry in twenty minutes.
- Nibble on bread and vegetables at those buffets and parties.
- Play some soft music—it suppresses your appetite.
- If you are stressed, walk it off, don't eat it off.

MIDNIGHT SUPPER FRITTATA

Makes 4 servings

1 onion, chopped fine
1 red pepper, seeded and slivered
Cooking spray
1 cup broccoli florets, blanched and drained
½ cup cubed cooked potatoes
1 sweet potato, cooked and cubed
6 egg whites
1 cup liquid egg substitute
¼ chopped parsley
⅓ cup shredded low-fat Cheddar cheese

Preheat the broiler.

In a large ovenproof skillet over medium heat, sauté the onion and pepper in a little cooking spray until softened, about 3 minutes. Add the broccoli and potatoes. Cook until heated through, about 1 minute.

In a medium bowl, whisk together the egg whites, egg substitute, and parsley.

Spread the vegetables evenly in the skillet and pour the egg mixture on top. Cover and cook over medium heat for 10 minutes, until the eggs are set.

Sprinkle the eggs with the Cheddar cheese and place under the broiler for 1 minute, until the cheese bubbles. Serve hot.

YOUTH NUTRIENTS PER SERVING

Calories	178
Calcium	200 mg
Vitamin C	77 mg
Beta-carotene	10,381 IU

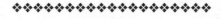

LAUGHTER IS HEALTHY

The secret of staying young is to live honestly, eat slowly, and lie about your age.
—LUCILLE BALL

SIXTY-SECOND CHEESECAKE

Makes 6 servings

15 ounces part skim milk ricotta cheese
2 tablespoons cocoa powder
5 packets Equal® sweetener
Dash of cinnamon
Dash of vanilla extract
½ cup raspberries

In a food processor or blender, process the cheese, cocoa powder, Equal®, cinnamon, and vanilla. Blend until smooth. Spoon into 6 of your fanciest dessert glasses and garnish each with a few raspberries.

YOUTH NUTRIENTS PER SERVING

Calories	110
Calcium	197 mg
Vitamin C	3 mg
Beta-carotene	320 IU

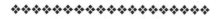

DO DAIRY FOR YOUNGER BONES

Surveys show that dairy products contribute 70 percent of the total available calcium in our diets. Check it out: How much do we really absorb?

26.7% of the calcium in whole milk
23.2% of the calcium in chocolate milk
25.5% of the calcium in yogurt
22.9% of the calcium in cheese
22% of the calcium in calcium carbonate

STRAWBERRY LOVERS SUNDAE

4 cups sliced strawberries
1 tablespoon sugar
½ teaspoon cinnamon
½ teaspoon nutmeg
3 cups nonfat, frozen strawberry yogurt

In a food processor or blender, process together 2 cups of the strawberries, the sugar, and the spices. Blend until the berries are mashed well. Divide the yogurt among 6 dessert dishes. Top with the remaining sliced strawberries and the blended sauce.

YOUTH NUTRIENTS PER SERVING

Calories	150
Calcium	173 mg
Vitamin C	57 mg
Beta-carotene	83 IU

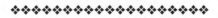

DESIGNER STRAWBERRIES

The USDA is beginning experiments to produce strawberries that contain more cancer-protecting antioxidants.

FLORIDA FRUIT SALAD

Makes 4 servings

2 grapefruits, peeled and sliced
4 oranges, peeled and sliced
4 kiwifruits, peeled and sliced
1 pint strawberries, washed and sliced

In a large glass bowl, toss all the fruit together and chill.

YOUTH NUTRIENTS PER SERVING

Calories	206
Calcium	154
Vitamin C	304 mg
Beta-carotene	800 IU

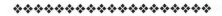

FLORIDA GRAPEFRUIT GET THE AHA OK

Florida grapefruit and grapefruit juice are the first fresh produce foods to receive the American Heart Association's heart check mark. Grapefruit is free of fat, cholesterol, and sodium and is loaded with the powerful antioxidant vitamin C

SCRUMPTIOUS FRUIT SALAD

Makes 6 servings

2 tablespoons lime juice
2 tablespoons lemon juice
¼ cup sugar
1 cantaloupe, peeled, seeded, and cut into chunks
½ honeydew melon, peeled, seeded, and cut into chunks
1 cup strawberries, hulled and cut in half
1 cup grapes
1 kiwifruit, peeled and cut into chunks

In a large glass bowl, combine the lime juice, lemon juice, and sugar and stir until the sugar is dissolved. Add the cut fruit and toss until the fruit is well coated. Cover and refrigerate until chilled and then serve.

YOUTH NUTRIENTS PER SERVING

Calories	138
Calcium	28 mg
Vitamin C	98 mg
Beta-carotene	2,974 IU

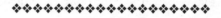

MELON MAGIC

A study at the University of Alabama School of Public Health found that women who included foods rich in beta-carotene, such as cantaloupe, in their daily diet reduced their risk of endometrial cancer by 27 percent.

HOT AND SWEET BAKED APPLES

Makes 4 servings

4 apples, washed and cored
¼ cup dried figs
¼ cup raisins
1 cup apple juice
1 teaspoon cinnamon

Preheat the oven to 350°F.

Peel the skin off each apple about a third of the way down from the stem end. Stuff each apple with a mixture of figs and raisins. Now place the apples in a shallow baking pan that has about an inch of water in it.

In a small bowl, combine the apple juice and cinnamon and pour the mixture over the apples. Cover and bake for about 30 to 40 minutes, basting often with the juices. Serve warm, right out of the oven, or cold.

YOUTH NUTRIENTS PER SERVING

Calories	171
Calcium	43 mg
Vitamin C	9 mg
Beta-carotene	93 IU

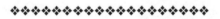

APPLES CAN LOWER CHOLESTEROL

French studies show that apples, rich in a soluble fiber called pectin, have the ability to radically reduce high cholesterol levels. Scientists believe that it is the combination of pectin and vitamin C, an antioxidant, that works the magic.

CLAFOUTI CAN-CAN STYLE

Makes 8 servings

Cooking spray
1 16½-ounce can cherries in light syrup
1⅔ cups skim milk
¾ cup all-purpose four
¾ cup sugar
1 teaspoon vanilla extract
¼ cup liquid egg substitute
1 egg white
Confectioners' sugar, for dusting
2⅔ cups low-fat vanilla frozen yogurt

Preheat the oven to 375°F. Spray an 8 x 8-inch baking dish with cooking spray. Spread the cherries evenly over the bottom and set aside.

In a large mixing bowl, combine the milk, flour, ½ cup sugar, vanilla, egg substitute, and egg white. Mix well with a wire whisk and pour the mixture over the cherries. Sprinkle with the remaining ¼ cup sugar and bake for 1½ to 2 hours, or until the mixture is set. Dust the top with confectioners' sugar. Serve warm and top each serving with ⅓ cup frozen yogurt.

YOUTH NUTRIENTS PER SERVING

Calories	286
Calcium	193 mg
Vitamin C	3 mg
Beta-carotene	1,035 IU

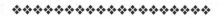

LOW-FAT AND SWEET

If you have a yen for something sweet, try some of these treats:

- rice cakes spread with all-fruit preserves
- dates stuffed with nonfat cream cheese
- raisins, dried apricots, dried figs, or dried apple slices

COUNTRY BREAD PUDDING

Makes 12 servings

Cooking spray
1 pound cinnamon-raisin English muffins, torn into small pieces
1 quart skim milk
¾ cup liquid egg substitute
1 cup sugar
1 tablespoon margarine, melted
Cinnamon, for sprinkling

Preheat the oven to 350°F. Lightly spray a 13 x 9 x 2-inch baking pan with cooking spray and set aside.

In a large bowl, combine the English muffins and the milk. Set aside and let them soak for about 10 minutes. Next, add the egg substitute, sugar, and melted margarine and mix together well. Pour the mixture into the baking pan and bake for 45 minutes to 1 hour, or until a knife inserted into the pudding comes out clean. Sprinkle with additional sugar and cinnamon. Serve warm.

YOUTH NUTRIENTS PER SERVING

Calories	207
Calcium	156 mg
Vitamin C	1 mg
Beta-carotene	545 IU

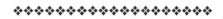

BOOST YOUR CALCIUM

By getting some of your daily calcium from nondairy sources, you increase your intake of other minerals such as boron. Why boron? Without it we just don't absorb calcium very well. And raisins are a terrific source of both calcium and boron.

BANANA RICE PUDDING

Makes 4 servings

Cooking spray
3 cups skim milk
1 cup rice
3 bananas, peeled and mashed
¼ cup raisins
1 teaspoon vanilla extract
Cinnamon, for sprinkling

Preheat the oven to 350°F. Spray a 1½-quart casserole lightly with the cooking spray.

In a large bowl, mix all the ingredients except the cinnamon together and pour into the casserole. Bake, stirring occasionally, for 1 to 1½ hours, or until the rice is tender. Sprinkle with cinnamon and serve warm.

Youth Nutrients Per Serving

Calories	339
Calcium	249 mg
Vitamin C	10 mg
Beta-carotene	445 IU

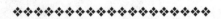

A LITTLE HUMOR

I have flabby thighs, but fortunately my stomach covers them.

—Joan Rivers

CLOUDS AND ANGEL CAKE

Makes 8 servings

1 banana, peeled and sliced
8 strawberries, hulled and sliced
1 kiwifruit, peeled and sliced
2 8-ounce containers low-fat vanilla yogurt
1 prepared angel food cake

In a medium bowl, mix together the fruit and yogurt until well blended.
Cut the cake into 8 slices and place each slice on a dessert plate. Top with
a mound of the fruit and yogurt mixture and serve.

YOUTH NUTRIENTS PER SERVING

Calories	304
Calcium	184 mg
Vitamin C	97 mg
Beta-carotene	10 IU

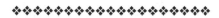

INTELLIGENT FOODS

Many manufacturers are adding important antioxidant nutrients to their regular
foods, everything from orange juice with added calcium to cereals with extra
beta-carotene. Great idea. How do we like it? We like it just fine.

Percentage of people consuming fortified foods daily

Cereal	40%
Orange juice	47%
Other fruit juices	38%
Fruit-flavored drinks	21%

ETERNAL COBBLER

Makes 8 servings

1 prepared angel food cake, cut into cubes
1 21-ounce can cherry pie filling
¼ teaspoon almond extract
2 pints vanilla frozen yogurt

Put the cake cubes in a microwave-safe casserole. In a small bowl, mix together the pie filling, extract, and ¼ cup water. Spoon the fruit mixture over the cake. Cover with plastic wrap and microwave on high for 5 minutes. Carefully remove the plastic wrap. Spoon the mixture onto 8 dessert plates and top with equal amounts of the vanilla frozen yogurt.

YOUTH NUTRIENTS PER SERVING

Calories	356
Calcium	167 mg
Vitamin C	3 mg
Beta-carotene	214 IU

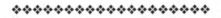

SOMETHING TO PONDER

By the time you are seventy-four you will have eaten the combined weight of six elephants.

—BOYD'S BOOK OF ODD FACTS

MELLOW-OUT BARS

Makes 36 servings

1 package yellow cake mix
1 16-ounce can pumpkin
¾ cup applesauce
¾ cup liquid egg substitute
½ teaspoon cinnamon
¼ teaspoon nutmeg
Cooking spray
2 tablespoons confectioners' sugar

Preheat the oven to 350°F.

In a large bowl, mix together the cake mix, pumpkin, applesauce, egg substitute, cinnamon, and nutmeg. Pour the batter into a 15 x 10 x 1-inch baking pan sprayed with cooking spray. Bake for 20 minutes, or until a toothpick inserted in the center comes out clean. Cool on a wire rack. When cool, dust with the confectioners' sugar.

YOUTH NUTRIENTS PER SERVING

Calories	76
Calcium	26 mg
Vitamin C	1 mg
Beta-carotene	2,893 IU

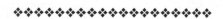

GREAT SUBSTITUTES

When baking substitute 2 ounces of soft tofu, mashed bananas, mashed potatoes, or applesauce for the eggs called for in most recipes.

SLENDER TRIFLES

Makes 8 servings

1 cup raspberries
1 cup blueberries
24 ounces strawberries, hulled and halved
½ cup sugar
½ prepared angel food cake, cut into chunks
1 8-ounce carton low-fat or nonfat vanilla yogurt

In a large bowl, mix together the fruit and sugar. Toss to coat well.
　　In a trifle bowl, alternate layers of the cake, yogurt, and fruit. Chill.

YOUTH NUTRIENTS PER SERVING

Calories	246
Calcium	97 mg
Vitamin C	40 mg
Beta-carotene	80 IU

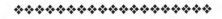

TREATS WITHOUT TOO MUCH GUILT

1 ounce taffy
3 small pieces of divinity
5 small meringue kisses
1 seven-inch candy cane
10 small gumdrops

DOG DAYS OF SUMMER FRUIT REFRESHER

Makes 8 servings

1 cup low-fat or nonfat strawberry yogurt
1 tablespoon orange juice
2 bananas, peeled and sliced
4 oranges, peeled and cut into chunks
1 grapefruit, peeled and cut into chunks
1 cup strawberries, hulled and quartered
1 cup seedless grapes

In a small bowl, combine the yogurt and orange juice and set aside.

In a large bowl, mix the fruit together. Pour the yogurt over the fruit and mix to coat. Chill.

YOUTH NUTRIENTS PER SERVING

Calories	116
Calcium	93 mg
Vitamin C	71 mg
Beta-carotene	281 IU

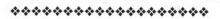

THE OLD "APPLE A DAY" WORKS

The British medical journal Lancet reported a study in which men who had a diet high in anti-aging nutrients, including lots of apples, were less likely to suffer a heart attack.

BE A GOOD SPORT DRINK

Makes 4 servings

½ cup sugar
½ cup hot water
¼ cup orange juice
¼ teaspoon salt

In a large pitcher, dissolve the sugar in the hot water. Add the orange juice, salt, and 3¼ cups of water and stir. Chill.

YOUTH NUTRIENTS PER SERVING

Calories	104
Calcium	7 mg
Vitamin C	8 mg
Beta-carotene	31 IU

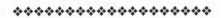

FRESH SQUEEZED O.J.

Orange juice has been shown to be effective against these killers: heart disease, high blood pressure, cancer, and rheumatism. It can also help you lose weight and give you a more youthful complexion.

STRAWBERRY-PEACHY SMOOTHIE

Makes 2 servings

½ cup fresh strawberries
1 fresh peach, sliced
1 banana
8 ounces tofu
2 cups orange juice

In a food processor or blender, process all the ingredients until smooth and creamy. Pour into tall glasses and serve.

YOUTH NUTRIENTS PER SERVING

Calories	280
Calcium	157 mg
Vitamin C	153 mg
Beta-carotene	881 IU

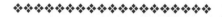

START EARLY

Experts recommend five servings a day of fruits and veggies. Here's how to make sure you get them all in and then some:

- Don't just have a glass of juice in the morning; add a piece of fruit, too.
- Make your morning muffins with applesauce instead of oil or margarine or butter.
- Snack on dried fruit, figs, and raisins.

HONG KONG SHAKE

Makes 2 servings

10 ounces tofu
1 banana
1 cup frozen strawberries

In a blender or food processor, combine all the ingredients and process until smooth. Pour into tall glasses and serve.

YOUTH NUTRIENTS PER SERVING

Calories	260
Calcium	166 mg
Vitamin C	56 mg
Beta-carotene	201 IU

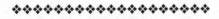

WANT TO LOSE FASTER?

- Turn off the TV and switch to relaxing music.
- Drink lots of water before, during, and after meals.
- Eat smaller meals more often.
- Before you put a snack in your mouth, take a five-minute walk—your craving will fade away.

ANTIOXIDANT COCKTAIL

Makes 2 servings

2 carrots
½ cup chopped parsley
½ head of cabbage
2 beets
1 red pepper
2 garlic cloves
½ cup broccoli florets

Put the vegetables through a juicer one at a time. Pour into glasses and serve at once.

YOUTH NUTRIENTS PER SERVING

Calories	183
Calcium	379 mg
Vitamin C	237 mg
Beta-carotene	26,519 IU

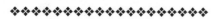

GIVE YOUR BODY A BREAK

Try a one-day fast to detox your system. (Drink lots of water.) You'll live longer and feel better.

BASIC YOUTH JUICE

Makes 1 serving

4 carrots
2 apples

Put the carrots and apples through a juicer and serve at once.

YOUTH NUTRIENTS PER SERVING

Calories	287
Calcium	97 mg
Vitamin C	43 mg
Beta-carotene	81,158 IU

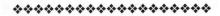

GETTING THE RIGHT TOOLS

A blender shakes up ingredients and blends them together.
A juicer extracts the juice and separates it from the pulp.

EDITA'S BONE-BUILDER DRINK

Makes 2 servings

1 cup shredded kale leaves
1 cup shredded collard greens
½ cup chopped parsley
3 carrots
1 apple

Put all the vegetables through a juicer. Pour into glasses and serve at once.

YOUTH NUTRIENTS PER SERVING

Calories	174
Calcium	326 mg
Vitamin C	94 mg
Beta-carotene	39,995 IU

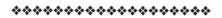

HIGH-CALCIUM VEGETABLES

Beet greens
Broccoli
Collard greens
Kale
Kohlrabi
Okra
Turnip greens

SALAD IN A GLASS

Makes 2 servings

½ cup broccoli florets
4 kale leaves
½ head of cabbage, cut into chunks
2 carrots
2 apples
¼ cup chopped parsley

Put all the ingredients into a juicer and process. Pour into glasses and serve at once.

YOUTH NUTRIENTS PER SERVING

Calories	264
Calcium	439 mg
Vitamin C	322 mg
Beta-carotene	36,878 IU

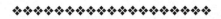

BEST BETS FOR BETA-CAROTENE JUICE

Apricots
Asparagus
Broccoli
Carrots
Dark leaf lettuce
Mangoes
Papayas
Pumpkins
Sweet potatoes
Winter squash

FAUX CHAMPAGNE

Makes 20 servings

1 32-ounce bottle club soda
1 32-ounce bottle ginger ale
1 24-ounce bottle white grape juice

Mix the club soda and ginger ale with the white grape juice in a fancy pitcher or punch bowl. Serve over ice.

YOUTH NUTRIENTS PER SERVING

Calories	36
Calcium	7 mg
Vitamin C	0
Beta-carotene	3 IU

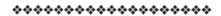

TIRED?

Drink more water. Eight glasses a day can help. Experts say that chronic dehydration leads to chronic fatigue.

DESIGNATED DRIVER MARGARITA

Makes 8 servings

1 6-ounce can frozen concentrate limeade
1 cup orange juice
1 cup unsweetened grapefruit juice
4 cups ice cubes

Put the limeade, orange juice, and grapefruit juice into a blender or food processor. Blend, adding the ice a few cubes at a time. Pour into glasses and serve at once.

YOUTH NUTRIENTS PER SERVING

Calories	65
Calcium	7 mg
Vitamin C	27 mg
Beta-carotene	64 IU

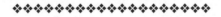

GET A LIFE . . . A LONGER LIFE

Estimates show that we swallow the following every single year:

- 300 cans of soda
- 5 pounds of potato chips
- 63 dozen donuts
- 50 pounds of cakes and cookies
- 20 gallons of ice cream

Thirty-three percent of us smoke and 10 percent are alcoholics.

"ALMOST SANGRIA"

Makes 6 servings

1 cup orange juice
2 cups apple juice
2 cups grape juice
1 orange, sliced
1 lemon, sliced
8 strawberries, washed, hulled, and cut in half
4 cups seltzer

In a large pitcher, stir together the orange juice, apple juice, and grape juice. Add the fruit. When well mixed, pour in the seltzer. Pour into glasses over ice and serve at once.

Youth Nutrients Per Serving

Calories	182
Calcium	66 mg
Vitamin C	160 mg
Beta-carotene	194 IU

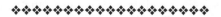

ALCOHOL: THE LIFE SHORTENER

Alcohol is responsible for over 100,000 deaths every year and 40 percent of all Americans have been in some kind of alcohol-related traffic accident, so moderation is the key.

BUBBLY BERRY BLUSH

Makes 8 servings

6 ounces frozen concentrate apple juice
12 ounces frozen concentrate cranberry cocktail
6 cups mineral water
1 lemon, sliced
8 strawberries, washed, hulled, and cut in half

Combine all the ingredients in a large pitcher or punch bowl and serve at once over ice.

YOUTH NUTRIENTS PER SERVING

Calories	138
Calcium	37 mg
Vitamin C	110 mg
Beta-carotene	59 IU

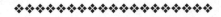

FRUIT = LOW-FAT

Check out these fruits and the percentage of their calories as fat:

Prunes	1%
Peaches	2%
Papayas	2%
Grapefruit	2%
Pineapple	3%
Cantaloupe	3%
Bananas	4%
Oranges	4%
Apricots	4%
Pears	5%
Lemons	7%
Blueberries	7%
Apples	8%
Strawberries	11%
Grapes	11%

GOLDEN SLUSH

Makes 4 servings

1 cantaloupe, peeled and cut into chunks
1 cup orange juice
¼ cup lemon juice
2 to 4 cups crushed ice

In a blender or food processor, process the cantaloupe, orange juice, and lemon juice with 2 cups of crushed ice. Add more ice if necessary to get a slushy consistency. Pour into glasses and serve at once.

Youth Nutrients Per Serving

Calories	78
Calcium	23 mg
Vitamin C	94 mg
Beta-carotene	4,431 IU

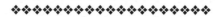

A REAL LIFE-EXTENDER

To get the most out of your cantaloupe, juice the skin as well as the pulp.

ROSY RED YOGURT SHAKE

Makes 4 servings

2 cups cranberry juice cocktail
2 8-ounce containers low-fat vanilla yogurt
2 oranges, peeled and chopped

Place half the ingredients in a blender or food processor and process until blended. Pour into a pitcher. Repeat with the rest of the ingredients. Place in the fridge and chill. Serve cold in tall glasses.

YOUTH NUTRIENTS PER SERVING

Calories	195
Calcium	244 mg
Vitamin C	92 mg
Beta-carotene	230 IU

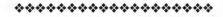

SMILE SOME MORE

Eat, drink, and be merry, for tomorrow we may diet.

TEXAS COCKTAIL

Makes 8 servings

1 48-ounce can vegetable juice cocktail
1 celery stalk
2 tablespoons lemon juice
2 teaspoons horseradish
1 tablespoon Worcestershire sauce
Dash of Tabasco sauce

Combine all the ingredients in a large pot. Set on low heat and simmer gently for 1 hour, until the flavors are combined. Discard the celery and ladle into cups. Serve hot.

YOUTH NUTRIENTS PER SERVING

Calories	36
Calcium	24 mg
Vitamin C	50 mg
Beta-carotene	2,000 IU

❖❖❖❖❖❖❖❖❖❖❖❖❖❖❖❖❖

BEST FITNESS EQUIPMENT

A pair of running shoes.

HALF AND HALF DRINK

Makes 2 servings

1 cup shredded carrots
8 ounces crushed pineapple in juice

Put the carrots and pineapple with ½ cup of water into a blender and blend at high speed. Pour through a strainer.

YOUTH NUTRIENTS PER SERVING

Calories	119
Calcium	49 mg
Vitamin C	22 mg
Beta-carotene	33,318 IU

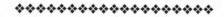

PINEAPPLE JUICE MORE THAN SWEET

Pineapple juice is high in vitamin C. Combined with carrots, this drink is a powerful fountain of youth.

SUPER COMBO

Makes 1 serving

4 ounces fresh carrot juice
3 ounces orange juice
Dash of Tabasco sauce

In a blender, combine all the ingredients and blend until well combined. Serve over ice.

YOUTH NUTRIENTS PER SERVING

Calories	83
Calcium	36 mg
Vitamin C	53 mg
Beta-carotene	29,380 IU

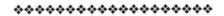

LAW OF THE MARKETPLACE

Change or perish . . . works for the food market, too.

PAPAYA SMOOTHIE

Makes 1 serving

6 ounces orange juice
1 tablespoon honey
1 frozen banana, sliced
½ papaya, peeled and cut into chunks

Put all the ingredients into a blender and process until well blended.

YOUTH NUTRIENTS PER SERVING

Calories	338
Calcium	44 mg
Vitamin C	141 mg
Beta-carotene	7,050 IU

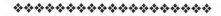

INDULGE

Indulge in "negative calorie" foods—foods that take more energy to burn than they themselves contain:

Cabbage
Apples
Grapes
Oranges
Tomatoes
Radishes

THANKSGIVING SHAKE

Makes 2 servings

1 8-ounce container apple juice
1 cup canned pumpkin
1 teaspoon cinnamon

Put all the ingredients into a blender and blend until smooth. Serve.

YOUTH NUTRIENTS PER SERVING

Calories	102
Calcium	33 mg
Vitamin C	51 mg
Beta-carotene	12,500 IU

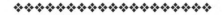

ANOTHER TIP ON HOW TO GET YOUR ANTIOXIDANTS

Pour apple, orange, grape, and cranberry juice into ice cube trays and freeze. Pop the juicy ice cubes into iced tea, fruit juices, and even water.

SUPERCHARGED TOMATO JUICE

Makes 1 serving

4 ounces tomato juice
3 ounces fresh carrot juice
Dash of Tabasco sauce

Pour all of the ingredients into a blender and blend for a minute until combined.

YOUTH NUTRIENTS PER SERVING

Calories	54
Calcium	32 mg
Vitamin C	19 mg
Beta-carotene	22,540 IU

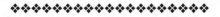

CHILI PEPPERS ARE "HOT" STUFF

Chili peppers are a wonderful source of antioxidants. Researchers have found that chilies reduce the risk of stroke and high cholesterol.

MILKSHAKE WITH A ZING

Makes 1 serving

1 cup buttermilk
1 ripe banana

Put the ingredients in a blender and process until smooth.

YOUTH NUTRIENTS PER SERVING

Calories	358
Calcium	281 mg
Vitamin C	12 mg
Beta-carotene	310 IU

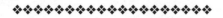

AIN'T IT THE TRUTH

As you get older, don't slow down—speed up. There's less time left.

—MALCOLM FORBES

GLOSSARY

Aerobic: A physical reaction that requires oxygen to release energy.

Alpha-tocopherol: The scientific name for vitamin E.

Alzheimer's disease: An incurable brain disorder characterized by memory loss and deterioration of mental abilities.

Antioxidants: A group of elements including vitamins E, C, and beta-carotene and the mineral calcium that fight free radicals.

Artery: A blood vessel that carries blood away from the heart and to the rest of the body.

Ascorbic acid: Scientific name for vitamin C.

Beta-carotene: An antioxidant found in fruits and vegetables that changes into vitamin A in our bodies.

Blood pressure: Measurement of the force of blood through blood vessels.

Bone: The part of the body that forms the skeleton. It is made of collagen and calcium phosphate.

Calcium: The most abundant mineral in our bodies. Our bones store 98 percent of it, and the remaining 2 percent circulates in our blood and tissues. It regulates our heart muscle, nerve impulses, and acts as an antioxidant fighting the aging effects of free radicals. Studies show that calcium is necessary for the prevention of osteoporosis, high blood pressure, and colon cancer.

Calorie: A unit that measures food energy.

Cancer: Uncontrolled growth of malignant cells.

Cardiovascular disease: A disease that affects the heart or circulatory system.

Carotene: A substance the body uses to make vitamin A. Carotene occurs naturally in many fruits and vegetables.

Carotenoids: This is the name given to over six hundred antioxidants that give color to fruits and vegetables and turn into vitamin A in our bodies.

Cholesterol: A substance that is produced in the liver as well as available through animal sources of food. It can build up in the wall of blood vessels, clogging them. There are two main kinds: HDL is "good" cholesterol, which vacuums out blood vessels. LDL is "bad" cholesterol, the one that clogs up blood vessels.

Collagen: A protein that provides the basic structure of bones, cartilage, and tissues.

Diabetes: A disease in which the body can't recognize or burn glucose (sugar) effectively. Glucose is needed for energy.

Dietary guidelines: National guidelines that recommend the amounts of various nutrients that should be taken by different age groups.

DNA (Deoxyribonucleic acid): The genetic blueprint in every one of our cells that regulates every single one of our characteristics and functions.

Electron: The name given to a unit of negative electrical energy. All atoms have some electrons. When an atom loses a vital electron it turns into a free radical.

Enzymes: Protein substances produced by cells that cause certain biochemical reactions in the body.

Estrogen: A female sex hormone produced by the ovaries that plays a large role in calcium absorption.

Fat soluble: Able to be dissolved in fat.

Free radical: The name given to an organic compound that has lost one of its electrons and is now unstable and can damage surrounding cells.

Genetic: Having to do with your genes—those elements that carry your entire blueprint.

Hayflick limit: A theory that states that cells can only divide fifty times before they die.

Hormones: Chemicals produced in glands that regulate certain body functions.

Hypertension: High blood pressure.

Immune system: An internal system that produces antibodies that fight bacteria, virus, and other invaders that can damage our bodies.

Life expectancy: A statistical estimate of how long you can be expected to live. Life expectancy has improved over the years and is now between seventy-five and eighty years.

Life span: A distinctive length of time that a human being is capable of remaining alive. For humans it is 120 years.

Metabolism: The total of all the processes going on in our bodies keeping us alive and functioning.

Nutrient: Chemical substance obtained from food that is essential for bodily functions.

Obesity: Weighing more than 20 percent over your desirable weight.

Overweight: Weighing between 10 and 20 percent more than your desirable weight.

Oxidation: This is a kind of circle of change having to do with oxygen. Atoms or molecules lose electrons while keeping us alive. This process then produces free radicals, which can damage our cells. Good examples of oxidation are rust and the browning of cut fruit.

RDA: Recommended Dietary Allowance or Recommended Daily Allowance, an estimate established by the Food and Nutrition Board of the National Research Council of the amounts of nutrients needed to prevent deficiencies in healthy persons.

Systolic pressure: Force of pressure when the heart muscle contracts.

USDA: United States Department of Agriculture.

Water soluble: Able to be dissolved in water.

Weight-bearing exercises: Exercises that cause mechanical stress on the bones and joints. Necessary for preventing osteoporosis.

INDEX